Pra
Melanie: Bird with a Brol

"Instructive, compassionate, beautiful..., ..., and truly inspirational— a must-read for every student and professional who works with families and children with disabilities and special health care needs."

—**Gail L. Ensher, Ed.D.,**
Professor of Early Childhood Special Education, Syracuse University; co-author,
Families, Infants, & Young Children at Risk: Pathways to Best Practice

"A must-read for anyone working with individuals with disabilities . . . a remarkable story told from the heart."

—**Sharon Vaughn, Ph.D.,**
University of Texas, Austin

"This book about a child and her mother, written with compassion and insight, is a "must read" text for healthcare professionals."

—**Karen Pape, M.D.,**
Medical Director, TASC Network, Toronto, Canada

"Anyone in the field of special needs and special education should read the book. . . . It gives us a nice glimpse into the life and mind of a mother of a child with special needs. I would recommend this book to anyone."

—**Janette Long,**
M.A. special education candidate, The Ohio State University

"This exquisitely written memoir shows the awesome responsibility professionals have in appreciating and reinforcing a parent's hopefulness. Beth's interactions with professionals show how hope can contribute to or undermine a parent's strength, a child's development, and the family's enthusiasm in engaging the arduous but always fulfilling journey."

—**Penny Camps, SLP,**
Child & Adolescent Center, Trinidad & Tobago

"This was not just a story for parents; it was both a professional and a life lesson . . . the unfiltered emotional descriptions throughout the story, the heartfelt poetry, and the photographs of Melanie truly inspired me."

—**Tara McCarthy,**
M.Ed. visual impairments candidate, The Ohio State University

"Shows what love, spirit, believing, and never giving up can do. Everyone should read it!"

—**Megan Rutschilling,**
M.Ed. visual impairments candidate, The Ohio State University

"Outstanding . . . As I read this book I cried, laughed, and felt fortunate that the author chose to share her daughter with us. What a beautiful story of strength, hope, determination, and love. I would certainly recommend this book for future classes."

—**Christina Woolard,**
M.A. intervention specialist candidate, The Ohio State University

"Beth Harry has shown great courage and progression of strength through her ability to recall the events of her daughter's life and create such an inspiring piece of work."

—**Jessica Ware,**
M.Ed. hearing impairments candidate, The Ohio State University

"This beautifully written memoir is deeply moving and insightful. With courage and honesty, this mother struggles through her darkest moments which unfold into a profound connection with her child."

—**Robert A. Naseef, Ph.D.,**
Psychologist, parent, author, *Special Children, Challenged Parents,*
co-editor, *Voices from the Spectrum*

Melanie

BIRD WITH A BROKEN WING

A Mother's Story

To: Cynthia
with best wishes
from Beryl Kenney

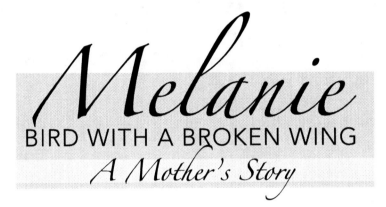

Melanie
BIRD WITH A BROKEN WING
A Mother's Story

by

Beth Harry, Ph.D.
University of Miami
Miami, Florida

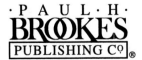

·P A U L·H·
BROOKES
PUBLISHING CO.®

Baltimore • London • Sydney

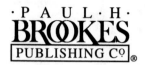

Paul H. Brookes Publishing Co.
Post Office Box 10624
Baltimore, Maryland 21285-0624
USA

www.brookespublishing.com

"Paul H. Brookes Publishing Co." is a registered trademark of
Paul H. Brookes Publishing Co., Inc.

Typeset by Broad Books, Baltimore, Maryland.
Manufactured in the United States of America by
Gasch Printing, Odenton, Maryland.

Library of Congress Cataloging-in-Publication Data
Harry, Beth.
   Melanie, bird with a broken wing : a mother's story / by Beth Harry.
     p.   cm.
   Includes bibliographical references.
   ISBN-13: 978-1-59857-113-4 (pbk.)
   ISBN-10: 1-59857-113-3 (pbk.)
   1. Harry, Melanie—Health.   2. Cerebral palsied children—United States—Biography.
   3. Cerebral palsied children—Family relationships.   I. Harry, Melanie. II. Title.

RJ496.C4H375   2010
618.92'8360092–dc22   [B]   2009052525

British Library Cataloguing in Publication data are available from the British Library.

2014   2013   2012   2011   2010

10   9   8   7   6   5   4   3   2   1

Contents

About the Author

Beth Harry, Ph.D., is a professor of special education at the University of Miami in Florida. A native of Jamaica, Beth graduated from St. Andrew High School in 1962 and went on to pursue her bachelor of arts and master's degrees at the University of Toronto and her doctorate at Syracuse University. Beth has been a teacher all of her adult life, including teaching English at the secondary and community college levels and special education at all levels. Beth's current work focuses on teaching and research related to disability, multicultural, and family issues. She lived in Trinidad for 12 years, where both her children—Melanie and Mark Teelucksingh—were born.

Acknowledgments

A warm thank you to all my friends and family members who encouraged me to move Melanie's story from its 27-year-old seat on my desk to the public eye. To authors who want to self-publish, I certainly recommend Xlibris for being efficient and reliable in assisting me to turning the manuscript into a "real" book. Furthermore, I thank the editors and designers at Paul H. Brookes Publishing Co. for taking it from there and giving *Melanie* the polished and professional look she deserves! I thank my colleagues at several universities who gave me wonderful feedback on the self-published version and immediately built it into their special education courses. I hope that with the help of Brookes that *Melanie* will find her way into the hearts and minds of many more parents and professionals. I thank my husband, Bernard Telson—for his loving support of the Melanie he never knew and of Mark—for whom he is always present.

*For Clive, Mark, Mercedes, and Mummy, in memory
of the beautiful Bird whose broken wing kept our feet on the
ground while her soaring spirit lifted us to the very tops of ourselves.*

*In telling this story, I celebrate the most important
lesson I learned from Melanie—that our natural inclination to resist
pain or unhappiness stands in contrast with the indescribable rewards of
loving in what Kahlil Gibran called "love's threshing-floor."*

My life has been easier, but emptier, without her.

Speak to Us of Love

When love beckons to you follow him,
Though his ways are hard and steep.
And when his wings enfold you yield to him
Though the sword hidden among his pinions may wound you.
And when he speaks to you believe in him,
Though his voice may shatter your dreams as the north wind lays waste the
  garden.

....

But if in your fear you would seek only love's peace and love's pleasure,
Then it is better for you that you cover your nakedness and pass out of love's
  threshing-floor,
Into the seasonless world where you shall laugh, but not all of your
  laughter, and weep, but not all of your tears.

—Kahlil Gibran, *The Prophet**

---

*Used by permission of Gibran National Committee, address: P.O. Box 116-5375,
Beirut, Lebanon; phone & fax (+961-) 396916; e-mail: K.gibran@cyberia.net.lb

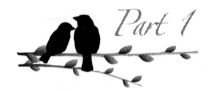

Chapter 1

WITH A WHIMPER

Clive said that his first moments of fear came when he saw the ash-gray color of her skin. My senses were not so sharp; having no idea of what a newborn baby should look like, I thought her strange but beautiful.

They said, "It's a girl!" But I felt no surprise, only a quiet fulfillment at receiving confirmation of what I had known all along. The doctor laid her on my stomach, and while he cut the cord that for 9 awesome months had bound her to me, I fondled the tiny down-covered head.

Suddenly, I realized that we were all waiting, and someone said something about a cry. After an interminable moment, there was a small sound. There was relief in the room, but I said, "That was a cry?"

And they said, "Yes, it's okay," and, I believe, some other reassuring comments. But my moment for fear had come, for I knew that my baby's first sound had been scarcely a whimper. The next shock was her weight. Four and a half pounds seemed very little for a full-term baby, but as I was wheeled out of the delivery room, I allowed myself to be comforted by the doctor's assurance that "the baby's fine." For the next hour or so, Clive and I talked. I have no recollection of what we said. Then he left, and I slept.

Later that night, on his return, it was Clive who said, "Where is she? I want to see her," and went directly to the nursery. I felt no inclination to see her, yet I do not recall being aware of harboring any specific fear or sense of her being in danger.

I can only surmise that the fear had gone underground, for the next afternoon, almost 24 hours after her birth, I had made no attempt to see my baby. My friend Ann arrived, her eyes filling with joyful tears at the news that I had my much-longed-for daughter. It was then that I finally roused myself and went to the nursery.

She was more beautiful than I had remembered, with no fat or baby wrinkles to hide or distort the delicately chiseled nose, mouth, and high wide cheekbones. Her face was exquisite, but around the tiny neck hung layers of thin loose skin such as one might expect in an old woman. Her body was perfectly formed and in proportion to the tiny head, and her skin, by then benefiting from the incubator's oxygen, a rich, dark brown.

She lay in her glass cubicle like a fragile china doll, her movements slight and her breathing imperceptible, and as I watched her, fear closed an icy hand around my heart. It was not until that night, however, that my fear became specific. I went to the nursery just as one of the midwives was trying to feed her, and I was taken aback at the sight of the diminutive little creature lying passively as the nurse tried to get drops of milk into her mouth from a tiny pipette. I watched, my terror rising, as I saw that the drops seemed to collect in her mouth and then dribble back out, and that, in a matter of minutes, the little forehead had taken on a purplish-gray hue. The nurse explained that the baby could not do without the artificial oxygen supply for more than a few minutes and put her back into the incubator, saying that she would have to try again later.

I left the nursery, moving as through a nightmare. All I knew was that my baby was frighteningly weak, could scarcely breathe by herself, could not suck, and apparently could not even swallow!

As I woke the next morning, I knew that fear had taken over; no longer a vague sense of something being wrong, it had hardened into a lump that seemed to sit at the very center of my being, and I knew then I was fearful for myself, fearful of the painful reality that I saw standing in front of me waiting to be grappled with. I could not do it! I could not cope with this!

I went to the nursery, and there she was, beautiful and still, and the words that filled my mind remain one of my most terrible memories: *You are beautiful, but if you're going to hang around and give me trouble, I'd rather you died.*

The words left my mind as quickly as they had entered, but I knew that they reflected a seed of resentment deep within me.

MELANIE

That was Wednesday morning, and I knew the pediatrician had been called in the night before, but we had, until then, been given no word of what might be wrong with the baby. We had decided to call her Melanie, but I kept referring to her as the baby. It was Clive who said, "Well, she's got a name now, let's use it!" And for him, from then on, she was Melanie. I knew only that she was not whom I had expected.

Finally I learned that my obstetrician would be coming to discuss the pediatrician's opinion with me, and he arrived that night, gentle and sober faced (up to that point he had been reassuring, almost jovial: "Baby's fine, just small"). His opening and parting words are the ones that remain with me verbatim. "Dr. McDowall's not happy about the baby," and "I know, it's worrying."

In between those two comments he talked, with a gentleness I had not expected from him, about the fact that she was underweight and underdeveloped for a full-term baby, with apparently immature respiratory and feeding systems, but that as she gained strength, these would probably improve. She was certainly weak, and it was too soon to attempt a prognosis. He spoke in a very general vein.

I can remember asking two questions: whether her brain might be damaged and whether there was danger of her becoming blind as a result of too much oxygen in the incubator. To the first, he replied that it was too soon to tell but that there could be that possibility. Insofar as she seemed generally underdeveloped, he said that this could possibly also be true of her brain development but that I should try not to worry about that yet. To the second question, he was very reassuring, explaining that he had just personally checked the oxygen-regulating system of the incubator, that it was correctly set, and that the oxygen-induced blindness of which I had heard was a phenomenon common to the early days of incubators before babies' oxygen requirements were properly understood.

Looking back, I realize that this conversation was, in fact, a preparation session for more painful news that would have to come later. It was an effective preparation, and it was kindly done.

The rest of that week is hazy in my memory. During the days I was exhausted and, at nights, wakeful in spite of the sedatives they gave me at bedtime. My bed was by the window, and I slept with the curtains open so as to see the outline of the hills whenever I opened my eyes. Their silhouette imprinted itself indelibly on my memory, and the words of the ancient psalmist filled my mind nightly as the hills became for me a symbol of the strength I would need in the days ahead: "I will lift up mine eyes unto the hills, from whence cometh my help, my help cometh from the Lord, who made Heaven and earth." (Psalm 121:1–2)

Chapter 3

EMPTY HANDS

I can think of no experience more disappointing than returning home empty-handed after giving birth to a baby. After 9 months of waiting, hoping, and fantasizing, a woman suddenly empty-bellied reaches aching arms outward to relieve the womb of its burden, and—nothing.

Of course this overstates my case: a woman whose baby has died is precisely in this situation. My baby was simply left behind for a while. Yet I felt robbed, cheated by my own body. The body I had always loved, enjoyed, and trusted to do its work efficiently and with ease had inexplicably let me down. I was to go home with an empty womb, empty hands, and a heart filled with fear.

This was what overwhelmed me on my last night in the maternity clinic—the next day I would go home without my baby. All week, I had been outwardly calm, but my tears were rising. Venus, the midwife in charge, came to sit with me and said, "We know you're brave, we can see that, but there's also a time for tears." It had been years since I had cried in someone's arms (like most adults, I had learned to prefer crying alone), but her kindness released me, and that night, I wept like a child in her mother's arms.

So on Saturday morning Clive came for me and we went home. Clive's niece, Paula, had come to stay with me for a few days, and I think she was taken aback to find me on the edge of panic.

I *was* on the edge of panic. Panda, whom Clive always referred to as "that hell of a mad dog," rushed to greet me and threw his paws against my stomach; I screamed in terror at the silly dog whose attempt at friendliness I perceived as a hostile threat to my disillusioned and vulnerable body.

For me, the most effective way of controlling fear has been to put it into words and to speak those words aloud, if only to myself. It is as if the spoken word gives form to a chaotic jumble of fears and offers a sense of control, however illusory, over a disordered world. Fortunately, I had people I felt I could talk to. Clive's niece, Paula, was one of the first people to whom I expressed what fears I was aware of, and I believe it was in an early conversation with her that I first expressed the feeling that I could cope with just about any problem my baby might have except mental retardation—the possibility of that seemed the most devastating of all.

In those early days, it was more difficult to talk to Clive about specific fears, probably for two reasons. First, I felt a reluctance to burden him further, knowing that he too was carrying his bundle of fears within him and struggling to keep them under control. Second, I respected *his* method of gaining control (almost opposite to mine), by appearing to keep his fears at bay until the extent of their reality becomes clear—that is, he preferred not to openly discuss fears while they were at the speculative state, but to wait until he knew exactly what he needed to be afraid of and then decide how to act. How different people can be from each other! For him, it was the possibility of action that brought a feeling of control; for me, it was the spoken awareness of whatever haunted me.

So in those days, Clive and I discussed mainly the practical, day-to-day issues of our situation, and there were many of these.

On the night I returned home, Clive went back to the maternity clinic to see how Melanie was and was told that tube feeding had been started since none of the normal methods of feeding

Melanie had worked so far. This first conjured up for me a vision of endless feet of tubing attached to a bedside drip, such as one sees on the medical soap operas on television, and which, at a later date I would actually see administered to Melanie. But the distinction was soon made between such intravenous tube feeding and this much simpler

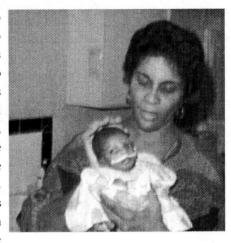

Beth and Melanie at 2 weeks with feeding tube

method of tube feeding of which I would also, at a later date, gain firsthand experience.

This turned out to be the insertion of a tiny polythene tube into the nose, down the esophagus, and into the stomach, the outer end of this tube reaching only as far as the baby's cheekbone and secured above her upper lip with a strip or two of tape. Nevertheless, it was a frightening sight—the strip of tape seeming to cover half the miniature face, and the very idea of such an artificial method of feeding emphasized the terrible inadequacy of this baby's feeding system.

But that night also brought cheering news, that although she was still being kept in the incubator for extra warmth, the artificial oxygen supply had been withdrawn, and Melanie was now breathing the same air as the rest of us! I was encouraged and went to sleep with my first recognizable touch of hope.

THE SWEET BIRD

The next morning, Sunday, marked the beginning of the most difficult period of my life up to that time: a period characterized by anxiety such as I had never imagined and an indecipherable mixture of hope and hopelessness.

Mornings were the worst—waking with a jolt into the cavern of anxiety that had become my world and surfacing only to encounter an onslaught of chaotic fears posing as reasonable questions: Was Melanie all right? What kind of night might she have had? Would they be able to take the tube out today? Would she have gained an ounce in weight? Would they say she might soon be able to come home? Then, fumbling my way through morning rituals in order to arrive at the only moment that mattered—seeing Melanie, seeing her alive and beautiful, and maybe, just maybe, a fraction stronger than the day before.

Besides visiting Melanie, there was one other activity that held any meaning for me—the struggle to produce breast milk for her. In the maternity clinic, my milk supply had started well, and I had been much encouraged by the midwives' emphasis on breast feeding and by their assurance that Melanie would receive whatever milk I could produce. So with the help of a little hand pump and two or three books on breast feeding, I embarked on a schedule of pumping and pumping and pumping!

Pump as I might, the milk supply dwindled from day to day, but I kept at it despite pessimistic comments from my obstetrician and active discouragement from the pediatrician (with whom up to then I conversed only by phone). I understood that there was little hope of the supply keeping up without the stimulation of the baby's sucking and in light of my state of anxiety (how I worked at relaxing!). What I did not understand, and I think the pediatrician did, was that the baby would probably never be able to suck well enough to stimulate an adequate supply.

But even if I had known this, I would have kept on pumping as though my life depended on it. I knew even then that I was doing this more for myself than for Melanie. There was the hope of contributing to her health, at least to the easing of her already poorly functioning bowels, but I knew that the amount of milk I was producing was not enough to be really effective. What I was really contributing to was my own sanity or, to be more precise, the maintenance of my self-image.

My self-confidence, normally pretty secure, had been dealt an unexpected blow: It had never occurred to me that I would be anything but a successful mother. True, conception had proved more difficult than I had expected, and after a hemorrhage at 10 weeks, my pregnancy had seemed shaky for a couple of months—the uterus growing very slowly, they said. But as soon as the baby started moving, I had put all the fears behind me and had plunged my whole being into the joy of carrying, protecting, and nourishing new life. I would be the natural mother—loving and confident—through one of life's most complex yet simple experiences. After all, wasn't I well equipped for motherhood? At 30, I felt myself moving surely into a phase of consolidation. My master's degree behind me, I was professionally and socially self-assured and inwardly self-accepting, and life seemed mine for the taking. I was in love with life and never doubted that life would forever be in love with me!

Now, in the space of a week, it was becoming evident that life, or my self, had let me down; things were not going according to plan, and a feeling of failure, an unfamiliar feeling for me, was beginning to set in. How could this be? Reproduction is one of life's givens, one of life's most basic activities; yet I had produced something less than perfect—a beautiful little weakling, a flawed and inadequate version of myself.

Surely the least I could do now was produce a modicum of nourishment for this little creature. And so I pumped and pumped!

Besides the presumably therapeutic value of this activity, there was the obvious fact that it gave me something to do. So I quickly established a daily routine; arriving at the clinic by 8:00 a.m., I would spend 2–4 hours in the nursery, admiring, holding, talking to, and inwardly weeping for my beautiful baby, Melanie. How the nurses put up with my continual presence in their small nursery for 8 weeks I cannot imagine. But they were unbelievably kind and encouraged me to develop confidence in my ability to handle Melanie and to relate to her, always providing me with a breast pump and bottle to express some milk while I was there.

Afternoons were spent at home, resting and doing my 3- to 4-hourly milk expression and reading anything I could get my hands on that related to childbirth, infant development, birth defects, parental attitudes, and so on. By 5:00 or 6:00 p.m., my anxiety level would have worked its way up again, and after a rushed supper Clive and I would set out to the clinic for anything from half an hour to 2 hours.

So my days were a rising and falling wave of anxiety and relief—anxiety that mounted steadily as long as I was away from Melanie and receded for as long as she was within my reach. There seemed to be no other concern in life but Melanie.

Clive was my rock from day to day, listening with patience to my recounting of every movement she had made, every sound, every ounce of milk consumed, and every ounce of weight gained or, as was often the case, lost. He was not as comfortable as I in the maternity clinic, surrounded by new mothers and smiling, chattering grandparents and fathers, and naturally was reluctant to take advantage of the privilege of spending time inside the nursery where there were normally only mothers, nurses, and newborn infants. So he spent his time there quietly watching Melanie through the nursery window and, whenever she was within earshot, whistling at her. It was this whistle that, some 7 months later, would finally elicit Melanie's first smile.

While Clive and I struggled within ourselves, Melanie fought to get a hold on life. Somehow, we never doubted that she would continue to live; yet her hold on life was tenuous, marginal, and as Clive kept saying, it was the quality of her life that we worried about. With the tube feeding, they were able to get enough milk into her to meet the requirements of life, but her body seemed able to make only minimal use of the nourishment, and it was some 3 weeks before she regained her birth weight after the usual initial loss of weight in the first week of life. She was weighed twice a week, and 1 or 2 ounces gained at midweek would often be lost by the weekend. Comparing this with what I knew was the normal pattern of weight gain for an infant (some 4–8 ounces a week), I knew that this could hardly be considered progress. It quickly became evident that there was no hope of breast or bottle feeding her, as her jaws were incredibly rigid and would clamp shut with the swiftness of a mouse trap at the slightest stimulation. Try as we might, we could get neither breast nor bottle into her mouth, and the nurse's one successful attempt at inserting her finger resulted in her being bitten so badly that she never tried again! The nurses told me that for such an infant, spoon feeding would be the only answer when the tube-feeding period was over.

Meanwhile, Melanie remained a beautiful but strange little baby, her strangeness impressing itself on me more and more every day. In a short time, her eyes were open, as bright and black as tiny ackee seeds, and with a fixed intensity of gaze that seemed out of place in a newborn baby. For Melanie's eyes never moved. It was not just that she did not follow objects; I knew that this skill could not be expected in an infant before about two months. The fact was that her eyes just *never* moved! I watched the other infants in the nursery and quickly discovered that, once open, their eyes continually darted from left to right—obviously in purposeless movement, but it was movement nonetheless.

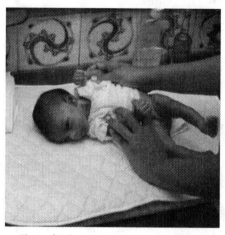

Photo of Melanie at 8 weeks (muscular rigidity)

Just as her eyes appeared fixed in one position, so did Melanie's limbs sometimes appeared to be fixed. This was by no means always so, as she certainly did move her limbs often, but I can recall times when she seemed almost to be stuck in a given position. On one occasion in particular, I watched her lying in the incubator, one arm flexed, the other stretched straight out to the side from the shoulder, head to one side, and eyes fixed directly ahead. The thought flashed through my mind that she looked like someone in a catatonic fit—a dramatic thought indeed, considering I had only a vague idea of the meaning of *catatonic*. Very much later, I would learn that this particular posture—the asymmetric tonic reflex (ATNR)—is in fact a primitive, reflexive position of the newborn that usually disappears within the first weeks of life. So the position itself was not abnormal, but the muscular rigidity I observed certainly was.

Another peculiar feature was a distinct tremor of the arms that was evident whenever Melanie moved them. This I also noticed in some of the other babies in the nursery, but in a much milder form.

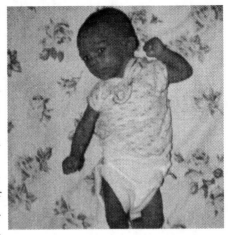

Photo of Melanie at 5 months (ATNR posture)

Perhaps the most striking idiosyncrasy of this little baby was her cry. The scarcely audible whimper she had uttered after birth had been succeeded by a cry greater in volume but very similar in quality. In fact, it was not what one normally considers a cry at all but was more like a tiny hooting sound one might expect from a bird. The main reason for this was that Melanie did not open her mouth to cry; with her jaws locked tightly, she simply pursed her lips and seemed to blow out, giving a somewhat high-pitched, gentle *oooooo, ooooo*.

From this cry, Melanie quickly derived two pet names: one, given her by a jovial nurse who always kept my spirits up, was Socialist, carrying the Trinidadian vernacular meaning of someone very polite and proper! The other name was given her by me, derived both from her cry and from the jerky birdlike quality of her movements—the Bird. So for me, within a few weeks, she was Bird, Birdie, Baby Bird—all in all, my beautiful, lovable, terrifying, beloved little Sweet Bird.

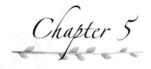

THE DREAM IS ME

Despite the consuming, overpowering love I felt for Melanie, it was not long before I had to admit to myself that my feelings were still not totally positive. The fears that had begun during the first week of her life still plagued me, and I knew that the only competitor Melanie would have was my own love of self.

I never doubted my love for her but often doubted my ability, even my willingness, to cope with the situation I found myself in. Was I prepared for the demands this child would make on me? For the repeated frustrations I knew lay ahead? For the hard work and dedication that would be required? Wouldn't it be so much simpler if she—the problem—would just go away, disappear, leave me alone?

I desperately wanted my baby to live, but I wanted also the joys of a normal motherhood, the reward of seeing a well-cared-for infant thrive and grow and develop. So far, I could see no promise, no hint of such rewards and was terrified by the thought of having to see myself so deprived.

And so I could not help knowing that on one level, I wanted her to die. The existence of this wish was thrust into my consciousness under two disguises: The first was an apparently innocent moment of fear and the second a dream.

I held Melanie for the first time when she was 7 or 8 days old. Until then, I had been merely a spectator, watching in awe as she was taken out of the incubator for feeding or changing. My sense of inadequacy was so great that it had not occurred to me to ask to hold her, and on Thursday, I believe it was the nurse who made the suggestion.

I held out my arms with a fearful eagerness. As the tiny bundle rested there, I was taken aback at her lightness and all at once overwhelmed by a sinking feeling in the pit of my stomach and a rush of weakness in my arms as though all their strength had suddenly drained away. It was as though I could not support such lightness. There was too little of her—no feeling of substance to command my support, to demand my strength. My muscles would surely turn to jelly, and I would drop her!

The moment passed. I emerged aware of a terrible tenseness in my arms—indeed throughout my body—and I knew that I had had to summon up every ounce of strength to support 4 pounds of life.

I realize that the momentary fear of dropping a baby is probably not an uncommon experience for new mothers. I have heard a number of mothers express fear of holding their new baby. This appears to me such an irrational fear that I cannot help suspecting that it conceals an element of desire: that it is, at least in part, a disguised desire to reject the baby and/or the awesome challenge and responsibility of motherhood.

Once more, I may be guilty of overstatement or excessive interpretation. I have no idea what psychologists would say on the subject, but I know that for me, the feeling of weakness, the feeling that the baby would inevitably fall, was very similar to the impulse to jump that often overcomes me when I look directly down from a very tall building. It is not a conscious wish to jump, but more like a feeling of powerlessness not to. Again, this is an experience that has been described by many people and that seems to me a kind of death wish.

This was how I interpreted the fear that overcame me when I first held Melanie: a death wish that arose not from lack of love, but from a sense of inadequacy and insecurity that said, "This is too much for me, I lack the strength, I cannot cope, I must be relieved of this burden, I must let it fall." This was my Gethsemane—"Let this cup pass from me." (Matthew 26:39)

For days I lived with an ever-present awareness of this wish, as usual, trying to gain control of it by forcing the feeling into words. The intensity of that moment of fear passed, but I remained nervous and uneasy in handling Melanie and found myself wondering if I would ever regain my confidence.

While I worked, largely unsuccessfully, at rationalizing away the fear that had taken up residence in me, that less-conscious part of the self that works at once more directly and more indirectly by presenting us with graphic yet symbolic versions of our conscious thoughts pushed me with unexpected force over the hurdle that was facing me.

Four or five mornings after holding Melanie for the first time, I awoke in terror from a dream—a nightmare—in which a small lizard in my house had turned into a crocodile that threatened me simply by virtue of its ugliness. I was terrified but pursued the creature with a large stick and discovered to my surprise that it was afraid of me. The chase continued through the house until eventually I had the intruder cornered and cowering before me.

This dream remained vivid in my mind all morning, and I struggled to make some sense of it. Looking for what in psychology is called the latent content of the dream, I tried to discover who or what might lie behind each of its figures. At first, I could think only of the possibility that the small lizard might represent my baby with whom I was dissatisfied and might soon come to hate and fear. In short, that the dream represented my rejection of Melanie.

But I knew this was the wrong interpretation: I was sufficiently in touch with my own feelings to know that this would be a gross distortion of the truth, for there was no question that I found her appealing both in her physical beauty and in her total innocence and helplessness. The fact that the creature in the dream began as a lizard made it clear that from the start my feelings toward it would be unequivocally hostile, for I have a horror of these creatures.

Some years before this, I had done some fairly intensive reading in the area of dream analysis and had actually developed some skill in interpreting my own dreams. The interest had faded over the years, and I had forgotten much of what I had learned. I recalled a paper I had written for a psychology course in which I subjected a dream of my own to three different methods of interpretation, using principles described by Freud, Jung, and the Gestalt therapist Fritz Perls. The theories of the first two had involved much detail, which now escaped me, and I could remember only some general principles. The Gestalt approach, however, has been impressed deeply on my mind because of its striking simplicity: The basic principle used by Perls in approaching a dream was simply this—The dream *is* me! I have created it, and therefore, every fragment of its structure represents a fragment of myself. One need look no further. As this approach came back to me, the meaning of the dream became instantly clear: *The dream is me. Therefore, the house is me. The "I" of the dream is me. The lizard-crocodile is me!*

The dream was very simply a representation of a battle within me. As is typical in tropical climates, the house lizard, a timid and harmless creature, was an unavoidable but unwelcome inhabitant of our home. His skill in keeping himself well hidden, especially during the day, was the only factor that enabled me to tolerate his presence. I could forget about him most of the time simply because he was seldom visible, but his hidden presence and his tendency to emerge at night lent a sinister aspect to his already unpleasant appearance. I was well aware, however, that my abhorrence of the little pest was totally irrational as I was obviously the stronger, larger, and more competent opponent.

And so my dream had presented me with this well-chosen symbol of one aspect of myself—an ever-present element of insecurity, which in favorable circumstances is seldom visible but whose appearance in a time of distress seems to constitute a threat out of all proportion to its size. On an unexpectedly dark night, the creature grows before my eyes into a crocodile, and I am forced to take up arms against him. His fearfulness of me gives me an advantage, and after a fierce pursuit I emerge the victor.

The victory, however, is a tenuous one for two reasons: First, the creature, though cornered in the end, does not return to his original size; he remains a crocodile instead of a lizard. Second, it is most significant that I have simply *cornered, not killed,* this unwelcome member of my house.

I knew then that any element of rejection of my baby, any fleeting desire for her death, was a monstrous outgrowth of my own human weakness. No matter how unacceptable I found it, this creature might be with me for some time, but I had already won the first round: I was aware of the presence of the beast, had gained some understanding of its nature, and could hold it captive in one corner of my house until such time as it could be eliminated altogether.

That I had made some headway was evident in the fact that on the very next day I held Melanie without fear. The sinking feeling in my stomach was gone, and I knew that I would be capable of doing whatever I had to do for her. In short, I would have the strength to be her mother.

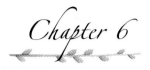

CRASHING

It was well that I was faced with this conflict between acceptance and rejection so early in the game (somewhere in the 3rd week of Melanie's life) since barely a week later, I was confronted with factual concerns that would distress me even further and require a truly accepting attitude.

The pediatrician had been keeping a close eye on Melanie, visiting her every 2 or 3 days, but the precise timing of his visits was irregular, and I had not yet managed to arrive at the maternity clinic at the same time as he. (Looking back, I suspect that this delay was an unrecognized aspect of my fear of hearing his diagnosis.) We had talked on the telephone several times, but naturally, I was anxious to meet him. So we finally arranged a specific time to meet at the clinic. It was an awkward time for Clive to be there, so I went alone.

Dr. McDowall arrived on time and turned out to be an older man, very conservative in dress and manner, with a dry, matter-of-fact tone of voice and a slowness of speech that kept me on tenterhooks throughout the conversation. I remember practically nothing of the first part of our discussion but assume that it related to Melanie's feeding and overall unsatisfactory progress. I remember being aware that he was leading up to something but had no idea what it would be. Rather suddenly he said, "Anyway, the thing I'm most concerned about right now is this—" and he demonstrated by pumping Melanie's arms up and down, bending them at the elbows, and then doing the same with her legs, explaining that in moving her limbs thus, one could feel an abnormal stiffness of the muscles. He directed me to do the exercise, then led me over to the next cot where he demonstrated the relative ease with which the neighboring infant's arms and legs could be bent. I followed his instructions and, with a pounding heart, observed that there was indeed a marked difference.

Taking a deep breath in an attempt to steady my voice, I said, "And how do you interpret this?"

With no hesitation and looking me straight in the eye, he said, "She has suffered brain damage." I felt something crash inside of me. I was intensely aware of the doctor's and nurse's eyes on my face and knew I could not break now. One more deep breath enabled me to respond. "You think so?" With a sinking heart, I heard him reply, "I am sure of it."

With a glance at the nurse, he then suggested that we should continue our discussion of this information outside of the nursery in a few minutes' time, after he had finished examining Melanie. I watched in a daze as he measured the circumference of her head, bent her head in different directions, tried to get his finger into her rather tightly closed fist, and tried to open her jaw. Then he turned her onto her stomach and watched as she struggled to lift her head. His tone displayed increased interest as he said, "Look, she's trying to lift up her head."

My hopes rose at the approval in his voice, and I could scarcely breathe in my anxiety to get out of the nursery where we could talk privately.

Outside, his manner, previously very professional and detached, seemed to soften slightly as he began a slow, deliberate explanation of his diagnosis. We must have sat there for some

20–30 minutes, and I cannot now imagine what words filled those minutes but vividly recall four or five points that, with the searing pain of a firebrand, scorched their way into my consciousness. I will record these points briefly.

The condition was, he said, what is known as cerebral palsy; I asked if this meant spastic. He explained that there were different kinds of cerebral palsy, of which the spastic type was one.

We must, he said, expect at the least that Melanie would suffer some degree of physical handicap, the extent of which could not then be guessed. Regarding her mental development, he said that this could quite possibly be perfectly normal, as this was often the case with people with cerebral palsy. I replied that I was aware of this as I had taught a student with cerebral palsy in junior high school in Toronto, and he had been a bright boy. He pointed out that increased emphasis on physical therapy made the prospects brighter for a person with physical disabilities.

Although any attempt at prognosis at this stage was impossible, he observed that there were, so far, two hopeful features of Melanie's development: 1) Her head circumference had increased in reasonable proportion to her size during the first month of her life, from which one could infer that her brain was, so far, developing within normal expectations, and 2) she was starting to try to lift her head not much later than the normal time.

In reply to my question as to the cause of her condition, he smiled slightly; clearly, he had been expecting the question. He replied that he felt quite sure it had originated with the bleeding I had experienced at 10 weeks and related further to the slow growth of my uterus in the subsequent month or so. He said that there was no evidence of damage suffered at birth and no reason to believe that there was any genetic factor at work.

These were the points of the conversation that remain with me, and the fact that it was not a monologue on the part of the doctor reflected partly his indication that he had both the time and the interest to respond to questions. It reflected also the intense need I felt to present myself as a rational, intelligent being well in control of my emotions and capable of coping with the situation. Why this was so important to me I cannot be sure. I imagine it was simply a result of my usual desire for things to go smoothly and reasonably and to be seen as a sensible, capable sort of person. But I could probably have accomplished this by simply receiving the information passively while maintaining my control. Instead, I was aware throughout the interview of an intense need to take an active part in the conversation, asking questions, making appropriate comments, and giving normal facial and gestural responses. I felt like something of a robot efficiently obeying the instructions of my control center. Whether or not the doctor saw me in this way I cannot guess, but this was how I saw myself.

I suppose that what I am really trying to describe is the discrepancy between the controlled performance I gave during that interview and the shattered, trembling, fragmented self that I knew existed at that very moment on some other level. On looking back, I realize that for a long time, perhaps a year, I continued to exist on these two planes—almost automatically acting in accordance with my habitual self-image yet constantly aware of the coexistence of a totally different and new self beneath the surface.

I remember that I told Clive that night what the pediatrician had said but cannot recall any part of his reply, which is unusual for me since I habitually can recall verbatim any important conversation I have had. I suspect that he said very little and do recall that from then on, his response, on the surface anyway, was characteristically different from mine. He seemed to regard this news as a piece of additional, almost peripheral information that could be shelved for the time being while we concentrated on pressing day-to-day problems that were demanding a solution, all of which, of course, revolved around Melanie's feeding difficulties—making the transition from tube to spoon feeding, increasing her milk intake, and getting her weight up to the required 5 pounds so she could come home.

This approach was in keeping with Clive's tendency to focus on the matters at hand and, in particular, on matters that we could do something about. Speculating, at that time, about the possible implications of a diagnosis of brain damage would be to him irrelevant and unhelpful. He subsequently explained that it would have made little difference in impact on him at that point whether Melanie had been diagnosed as having an acute liver ailment or a hole in the heart since it had been obvious from the beginning that something was seriously wrong, and the long-term implications of any given illness were pale in comparison to the immediate problems—would she thrive, and would she establish a firm hold on life?

In this way, Clive was able to maintain a practical, *first things first* attitude. In a way, I suppose I did too, insofar as I was able to continue doing whatever had to be done, and I certainly had to attend to Melanie's feeding problem since spoon feeding was about to be started, and the nurses insisted I be involved from the start. But beneath the apparently efficient functioning of my outer self, I was devastated by the diagnosis: A hole in the heart would have been far easier for me to cope with. I had been given news more unacceptable to me than any I could have imagined.

GARGLING

The news of the diagnosis came to me just at the time when Melanie's transition from tube to spoon feeding had been initiated; my active participation was now required, and this new phase was the first concrete sign of progress in her feeding.

Venus, the midwife in charge of the maternity clinic, despite the tremendous demands on her time and energy, took on the task of teaching me to spoon feed Melanie, which turned out to be not at all a simple procedure. Each step was a problem: first, to get Melanie to open her tightly pursed lips, then to relax the traplike jaw just enough to get the tip of the spoon in, then to get her to relax her tongue so that the spoon could be placed on the top instead of below it, thus allowing the milk to go down her throat instead of over her lips and down her chin. But these were preliminary difficulties that mainly required Melanie's growing accustomed to the unfamiliar oral stimulation and our handling her gently but firmly. She was soon allowing the spoon in quite willingly, though the proper positioning of her tongue took her longer to learn.

Within a few days, however, as the amount of milk we were offering her was increased, a new and, at first, baffling problem arose. After the first ounce or so of milk, we would hear the beginning of a rattling noise in her throat; this would rapidly increase until Melanie—her whole body tense, neck and shoulders arched tautly—was making a noise in her throat that the nurses and I could only describe as gargling. It was exactly like someone gargling a liquid in the throat but becoming short of breath and exhausted by the effort. The nurses seemed to be as baffled as I was, and we began assuming that perhaps as a result of the tube feeding she had developed an excessive amount of mucus in her throat and that this was the source of the trouble.

It so happened that at this time, our pediatrician was out of town for a few days, so the nurses contacted another doctor, and there was talk of trying antihistamines to dry up the mucus and of whether there might even be some throat infection that should be treated with antibiotics. I cannot recall which medication was finally tried, but it seemed to make no difference, and for several days, it was a matter of giving Melanie a rest (the gargling would usually fade away within half an hour or so) or sometimes trying to clear her throat by means of suction apparatus. The latter procedure seemed to help sometimes, but we were not sure whether what was coming up was really mucus.

As soon as our regular pediatrician returned, I spoke to him on the phone and described the problem. I recall his immediate response: "Mucus? Is it mucus or milk? It might be that she's not swallowing the milk."

My own inner response to this comment was sheer incredulity; of course she was swallowing the milk! She would do fine for an ounce or so, and then this collection of mucus would start to interfere. It had to be mucus; it would start off sounding just like the rattle on the chest of a person with a bad cold (it could even be heard sometimes in her sleep) and would gradually come to sound more like active gargling. In any case, we agreed that he would come to investigate the problem that evening.

I was disappointed that he could not be there to actually see her being fed, but after suctioning her throat and examining the fluid that came up, he seemed satisfied that there was little more than a normal amount of mucus and restated quite firmly his original suspicion that what was collecting in Melanie's throat after a short period of feeding was, very simply, the milk she was supposed to have been swallowing. In other words, this helpless little creature could not perform or, at least, could not perform for very long one of the most basic survival functions—she could not swallow.

It is true that this had appeared to be the case in the nurses' early attempts to feed her with a pipette, but I had not really given that particular feature much thought as I had assumed that it was probably a part of her overall weakness at birth. This feature had, of course, not shown up during the tube-feeding period, which was a purely passive procedure for Melanie. The pediatrician now explained that Melanie's inability to suck or swallow was an indisputable sign of damage to at least one part of the brain, in fact to the most primitive part that controls automatic, reflexive responses with which babies, indeed almost all creatures, are equipped at birth and do not need to be taught. His advice was that we should continue to try to spoon feed her, since the process of swallowing would have to be learned through constant practice. The ability to suck, he felt, might also be learned and might be facilitated by the use of a special bottle known as a Belcroy bottle or its newer version known as a Brecht feeder.

With this suggestion, we began our search for what I hoped might be an answer to at least part of Melanie's feeding problem; I hoped that if she could develop some sucking reflex, this might stimulate the swallowing reflex and get the whole system on the move. The pediatrician himself was unable to help us in the search for a bottle, and his contacts at the hospital could not recall having seen a Belcroy bottle for many years. The nurses caring for Melanie knew of the bottle but had access to none. We got in touch with all the people we could think of in Trinidad who might be able to help, including a friend who owned a hospital supplies firm, but with no luck.

Finally, in desperation, we sent off cables to my cousin Bruce, a doctor who was at the time resident in England, and to my mother in Jamaica. Although I think the Belcroy bottle was originally a British invention, my cousin discovered that it seemed to be completely off the market there. My mother had better luck: through my father's medical practice, she had years of contact with the medical profession and knew all the right people to ask in Jamaica. We sent her the cable on a Tuesday, and on Thursday night the precious little package arrived courtesy of an airline pilot who was a friend of a friend of Mummy's. The bottle was a version of the Belcroy, with a different name but based on the same principle. It had two special features, the main one being a little rubber squirter on one end, which when pressed would simply squeeze the milk into the mouth of the baby who could not pull for herself and, at the other end, a small elongated and unusually soft feeding nipple, again intended to facilitate a baby with a very weak sucking action.

The nurses agreed to try the new bottle with Melanie on Friday evening, and I went to the maternity clinic all excited and full of hope for new developments. Of course, it was a problem just getting the nipple into the Little Bird's mouth, but this was eventually accomplished. The nurse and I both felt that if Melanie could squeeze the milk out for herself, this would be better than us squirting it in, and we proceeded on this basis. It was soon evident, however, that Melanie was doing nothing at all with the nipple, so we decided to try squeezing it in as a start, in the hope that after getting used to the feeling of the nipple in her mouth, she would eventually try to suck for herself. So we squirted as gently as we could, and Melanie seemed to be swallowing for a while.

The rattling in her throat soon started, however, and I think that in our zeal to make the new bottle work, we pushed her a little further than we normally would have. Soon she was into a severe

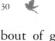

bout of gargling, and it dawned on us that she was terribly exhausted and breathing very rapidly and with difficulty. We soothed her as best we could and put her down in her cot to rest. I stood looking at her for several minutes before leaving. I had not seen her look so weak since her first days of life, and her extreme vulnerability terrified me.

My fear proved well founded: the next morning I arrived at the clinic to see, to my horror, the hated strips of tape once more across her upper lip, and the little feeding tube peeping out above it. This was one of my few moments of loss of control while actually in the nursery; tears rushed to my eyes, and all I felt was a massive sense of failure. Melanie had taken a step backward, and it seemed more than I could bear. The head nurse stood beside me, comforting but firm, explaining that Melanie was obviously not ready for the bottle yet and in fact was doing so poorly on the spoon feeding that she had actually lost a little weight. She had been so overtired after her efforts on the previous night that they had had to put her back in the incubator for the night with a supply of extra oxygen to help her breathing. They felt that she definitely needed a rest and should be tube fed for a few days to spare her the exertion of trying to help herself and give her a chance to regain some weight and strength.

This meant that Melanie's excursion into the realm of normal feeding had lasted only about 5 or 6 days, and here she was again, totally dependent on an invention of modern science. I was heartbroken and more fearful than ever—where was this going to end? Indeed, if I could have seen into the future and had any idea of the number of times I would ask myself that question, I would not have had the strength to go on. Fortunately, there were the everyday facts to face, and these offered some limits to my imagination, which otherwise would have tortured me with horrifying visions of the future.

The sum of the matter presently at hand was that Melanie was kept on the tube for about 3 more days before resuming attempts at spoon feeding, at which point I tried to be present to give her most of these feedings in order to gain confidence and skill in handling her. She did seem a bit stronger after the rest period on the tube, and the difficulty in swallowing seemed a little improved. She was now able to swallow perhaps up to 2 ounces before the gargling set in, and we were aiming at an intake of 13–15 ounces a day. But with six feedings a day and her ability to take only 2 ounces at a time, she was still falling below the mark.

We persisted, however, and after 2 or 3 days, our hopes were sufficiently raised for the big, long-buried question in our hearts to be brought to the fore: when might she come home? For the first 4 weeks of her life, we had scarcely dared to ask the question. The onset of spoon feeding had seemed to present the beginning of a hope in that direction; the resumption of tube feeding had once more buried the thought, and finally, here we were in her 6th week of life seeing a real glimmer of the possibility of having her at home.

The glimmer was transformed into a light more suddenly than we expected. It seemed to occur as a real possibility to us and to the nurses at the time, and they expressed the view that I was quite capable of coping with the feeding and would only learn more by caring for her full time. Also, as they said, there was little to be medically done for Melanie now—it was a matter of good care and, above all, patience. In other words, all we could do was care for her to the best of our ability and leave the rest to time. The doctors agreed that they had done as much as could medically be done and that now it was up to us.

We agreed that Melanie would come home that Thursday, October 30th, 1975.

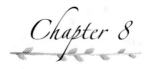
CHOKING

Much has been written about the distressing but perfectly understandable ambivalence of mothers upon the delayed homecoming of a newborn infant. The mother may become accustomed to the idea of a shared rather than a total responsibility for the child's care and is unsure of her ability or even her willingness to assume such a burden. She has become somewhat dependent on the well-trained institutional staff who have cared for her child thus far and cannot imagine doing the job as well as they did.

By the time of Melanie's homecoming, I had already read reports of such mixed feelings, but fortunately I did not experience them. I wanted her at home without reservation; I had found the hours of separation from her so agonizing that I was sure the difficulties of caring for her 24 hours a day could not possibly be harder to bear. Besides, I felt that, with her to care for, I would have no time for the tortuous imaginings and fears that habitually haunted me when I was away from her.

The truth of this expectation hit Clive and me with full force within a day or 2 of Melanie's arrival at home. One can appreciate the extreme patience of the staff at the maternity clinic when I say that it took, on average, 1 hour to feed Melanie 2 ounces of milk by spoon if she was doing fairly well. In a bad session, where the choking and gargling set in early, it would often take half an hour to give her *half an ounce.* The day she came home, I started keeping a diary of her feedings, noting the length of time and the amount taken as well as commenting on the ease or difficulty of the feeding. Looking over this diary now, I am astounded to see notes like 2:30–3:00 a.m.—½ oz; 6:15–7:45 a.m.—2¼ oz, and so forth, and occasionally, something as good as 1:30–2:30 p.m.—2½ oz!

But it was not really the length of feeding time that was exhausting and frustrating. It was the emotional energy required to hold on my lap a little mite weighing less than 5 pounds and gently but firmly pour down her throat spoonful after spoonful of milk in the hope that it was going down (for I still could not always tell if she had swallowed it); in the *hope* that she would recover from the recurring fits of choking and coughing (that she *did* cough was a blessing!); in the *hope* that I was not overtiring her in offering her just another quarter of an ounce; and then trying to maintain my own sense of calm while attempting to soothe and calm her during and after a fit of gargling and trying to bring some relaxation to the tense, tautly stretched, and stiffened little body.

The last problem was perhaps the worst: Melanie was, much of the time, like a little tight-rope across which one could discern constant undulations and fluctuations. To describe her as restless would be a ridiculous understatement, and her habit of stiffening and arching neck and shoulders and thrusting her head backward made her uncomfortable to hold and often distressing to look at. Along with her still rather faint cry, she made constant fussing or fretting noises much of the time and had developed a habit of frowning that made her seem the oldest, most unhappy little baby possible. She seldom slept for more than 5 minutes at a time during the day, and though she slept fairly well at night, the midnight feedings were often so slow that we would be up for 2 exhausting hours working at 2 ounces of milk.

We struggled along like this for about 5 days with little change for better or worse. On the 6th day, a new problem arose— Melanie started vomiting. She would appear to be swallowing quite well, then all of a sudden, up it all came. The milk she brought up looked as fresh as when it went in, with no sign of having been partially digested. This continued at most feedings all of that Wednesday and Thursday, and the scales were already showing a loss of a few ounces.

Then on Thursday night, we had a terrible scare. I had put Melanie down in her cot in our room and left her for a few minutes. On going to check her, I was horrified to see her lying on her back (I had put her on her side as I had been taught to do), eyes bulging, gasping for breath. I grabbed her, started hitting her on the back, and when this did not help, I turned her upside down and pounded for dear life. She was still gasping when we rushed in to the car and set out for the maternity clinic. After a minute or two in the car, there came the faintest cry, and we realized that the danger was over; she had finally caught her breath and was soon crying quite steadily in what seemed to be fright. At the clinic, the nurse on duty was very kind and, after checking her thoroughly, assured us she was fine. We could only assume that she must have choked on her vomit, although there was no sign of anything having been regurgitated.

We were thoroughly shaken by this episode and made our way to the pediatrician's office the next morning. I took her formula and, having described the various aspects of the problem to him, proceeded to feed her so he could see for himself. After perhaps 6 or 7 spoonfuls, the doctor said simply, "She's not swallowing." I said I thought she was, and he said, "No, she's not." The very next minute, up came a gush of milk. The doctor pointed out that what was happening was that the milk was simply collecting in her throat and then being ejected.

After a few minutes discussion, the doctor reached for the telephone, saying that he would ask the maternity clinic if they would take Melanie back for a couple of weeks. He felt that perhaps 2 more weeks on the tube feeding would give the problem time to improve as she gained weight and strength. My immediate reaction was "NO!" I could not go through that again. After 2 months of waiting, how could I endure the disappointment of such an anticlimax? Only 6 days at home and we must lose her again! Clive was more inclined toward the doctor's view, however, and we finally decided to watch her for another day and see what would happen. This was the final word as we left the doctor's office, but on the way home, after discussing the problem over and over, I realized I was simply being stubborn. Trying to prove that she could remain at home even though she was keeping nothing down and losing weight would be pointless. I wanted so much to see progress and could only see her return to the maternity clinic as a regression. I could not see then that this was only the beginning of a pattern that it would take me almost 2 years to recognize and accept: that regression in Melanie's development would not necessarily mean failure but rather an essential step in her path to progress.

So that day we drove home, collected Melanie's clothing, and went back to the clinic. We told the nurse on duty what had happened and suggested she telephone the doctor to check. Having done so, she very kindly agreed to keep Melanie although this was not normally their policy because this was a maternity center; once a baby had left, they would not usually take her back.

We thanked her, and within half an hour we were on our way back home, once more empty-handed.

Chapter 9

VOMITING

By the time of Melanie's second homecoming 2 weeks later, I was better prepared than I had been for the first. By this I mean that I was developing a habit of preparing myself for disappointment while at the same time trying to hang on to my natural optimism. If I was to maintain some measure of equilibrium, it would be essential for me to learn to tread the fine line between optimism and pessimism. Pessimism, I felt, would have to serve as a defense mechanism for myself; optimism, as a defense mechanism for Melanie. If I hoped for too much, I would be constantly disappointed, but if I hoped too little, I would be incapable of helping Melanie.

So 2 weeks later she came home for good. The doctor's guess had been partially right, and in fact, upon the resumption of spoon feeding, the nurses found that the gargling response had almost disappeared. It had been replaced, however, with consistent regurgitation of a substantial amount of the food.

Melanie had made progress: whenever her swallowing mechanism failed to work, the milk, instead of staying in her throat and producing the gargling effect we had become accustomed to, would now be ejected. *What painful progress! She had learned to vomit rather than to choke.*

Melanie was, by then, weighing close to 5 pounds, and despite the tiny frame she was surprisingly strong and quite unlike the limp little newborn I had held for the first time some 8 weeks before. Her movements were noticeably stiff, the tremor in her arms still visible though much reduced, and there was

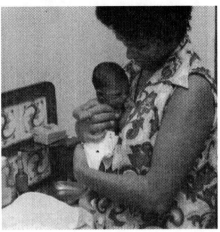

Eight weeks: home at last

now a tremor in her jaw, which occurred quite often during feeding and could actually be heard—something like the chattering of teeth. The tendency to arch her head backward was still marked, and her hands were constantly held in a tight fist. She moved a lot when held, and anyone holding her would invariably comment on her strength.

But of all Melanie's physical features, the one that now bothered me most was her apparent inability to use, or, more precisely, to *move* her eyes. When I would come into her line of vision, she would appear to be looking straight at me, and I had the distinct feeling that she was seeing me. But if I moved off to one side, her eyes would remain fixed in the same position and with the same apparent intensity of gaze. Her gaze did not seem vacant to me; on the contrary, I thought it quite attentive, but then her lack of attempt to follow me made me wonder if in fact she was seeing at all.

The terrible thought that she might be blind haunted me for weeks, and on the day of our first visit to the pediatrician's office,

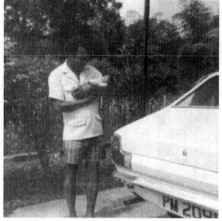

At home with Daddy

I told him of my fear. As I spoon fed her, he sat beside me and watched, and my heart leapt in gratitude as he agreed with my own instinctive impression. As she gazed steadily at me, he said, "She *is* seeing," and then, "Yes, she is attending." When I pointed out that if I moved out of her line of vision, she made no attempt to follow, he said that the ability to follow by moving the eyes would not be expected in a baby of 7 weeks, especially considering her slow start.

I was reassured by his seeming so sure that she had vision but was still deeply worried because I knew that in my very close and constant observation of her, I had never once seen her move those bright black eyes. It was true that they would sometimes be in different positions, but always it seemed to me that it was her head that had moved and never her eyes. For example, if she turned her head to the right, her eyeballs, which had been centered, would then be seen to be in the left corners of both eyes. If she turned her head to the left, they would be seen in the right corners. What was really strange was that bending her head down made her eyes appear to roll upward, and lifting her head up made them appear to roll downward. As I saw it, the fact was that her eyeballs just never moved; I tried it myself and found that if I centered my gaze on an object and bent my head down without letting my eyes move from the object, then I would, of course, appear to be peering upward, and so on.

Perhaps the only aspect of Melanie's development that was not worrying was her hearing. From the early weeks in the maternity clinic, I was sure that she was responding to my voice. If she was lying in her cot, my speaking to her always produced some kind of change in her behavior. If she was moving when I spoke, she would immediately freeze. If still, she would move. Sometimes the response would be to stop crying or to start. So she was not only hearing, but she was also responding.

Her general beha- vior was still distressing —her fretfulness and her constant arching, tens- ing, and choking. There was simply nothing relaxed or relaxing about Melanie. My parents had come the day before her return home, and one of my mother's first obser- vations was that she was constantly frowning or "scowling" as Mummy

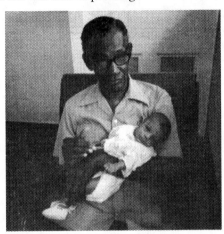

At home with Papa (Grandfather)

put it. This was a new development and certainly was distressing to see. I had to admit to myself that much of her waking time, my beautiful Little Bird looked like a bad-tempered, irritable old woman!

Nevertheless, Melanie was home at last, and her care, her development, her life, were totally in our hands.

Chapter 10

IN OUR HANDS

Let me step back for a few moments.

Remembering my keen anticipation of taking full responsibility for the care of my precious Little Bird, I am led to reflect on who we were—Clive and I—as individuals and as a family. We were, above all, a couple who had come to adulthood and to our marriage from the experience of solid and supportive family networks. I believe this was a huge force in the way we responded to Melanie's needs.

For Clive, as the third in a family of 11 siblings, a sense of responsibility to the group was balanced by a powerful individuality easily seen in his assurance about his own ideas and his lack of concern for the social prejudices so common in small communities such as our Caribbean islands. Growing up in Trinidad, a key part of his social identity reflected the society's construction of race—an inclusive approach by which all racial mixtures are taken into account. Clive would be described as a *dougla*—a mixture of Indian and African origins very common in Trinidad's multiracial society. My own racial identity included both the African and European origins of my parents, so in Trinidad I was most often referred to as *red*, while in Jamaica, most people would call me *brown skinned.* But Clive was notably unimpressed either by racial identity or social status. Indeed, there was a meticulous self-containment about him that hinted at aloofness, but those who knew him well understood his reserve as a confidence that was more internal than social—a quiet respect for himself and for others that placed him somehow above the fray. At the time of his death, 33 years after Melanie's birth, his sister Vilma wrote these words to be read at his farewell service:

> Clive was the embodiment of Christian values—charity, forgiveness, mercy, kindness, generosity to those less fortunate than himself. He never discriminated on the basis of class or background. Though he was never inspired to go to church regularly or to read the Bible carefully, he somehow emanated the Christian values we all wish to learn. Quiet, unassuming, and gentle, he had qualities that could be mistaken for weakness, until you tried to dislodge him from a carefully thought-out position. A hero without the noise and fanfare. A man whose life was inspirational to all of us.

Vilma's reference to religion reminded me also of where Clive and I first met. It was in our first-year philosophy class at the University of Toronto—a class that was to have a profound impact on both of us in terms of cementing a natural skepticism that we shared toward formalized versions of spirituality. Clive had been raised Roman Catholic and I, Anglican, but although attending church was a required part of growing up, neither of our families was rigid in its beliefs. In my own family, my father's education as a physician and his openness to a range of ideas afforded my two brothers and me a sense of freedom to determine our own paths. So I would say that our families' unquestioned assumption of the verity of Christian doctrine and principles was tempered by a strong pragmatism that had shaped our values and allowed us to follow our own interpretations of life's gifts and challenges. From the early years of our relationship, Clive and I acknowledged that we were both agnostic in relation to religion, yet continued to be rooted in the values and ritual language of one of the world's most powerful belief systems.

I refer to the ritual language of Christianity with a sense of nostalgia and longing. The poetry of the Bible and, in particular of the psalms, was an ingrained part of my education at St. Andrew High School, which was in those days one of the most sought-after girls' schools in my native Jamaica. Our school, run by a combined board of the Methodist and Presbyterian churches, provided an education deeply rooted in traditional British curricula and practices, which included daily prayers and religious readings and hymns. My peers and I knew most of the hymn book by heart and would learn the psalms as much through repetition as through occasional punishments that required much copying and memorizing! This education offered me a flawless preparation for pursuit of my bachelor's degree at Trinity College, the Anglican enclave of the University of Toronto's massive, cosmopolitan educational system. Clive had received the equivalent education at St. Mary's College, Trinidad's most prestigious Catholic, all-male high school.

Explaining my deep connection to Christian values and concepts helps me to interpret my reaction to the challenges Melanie brought me. By the time of her birth I had come to regard the beliefs of Christianity as an overarching metaphor for our human sense of the importance of our lives. For me, personally, it is difficult to imagine that, given the challenges of human life as a whole, my own life should be important enough for even an omniscient creator to attend to. I believe that the creative force behind the universe is expressed in all its aspects and that human life, as only one of those aspects, cannot be interpreted in terms of individual wishes and needs; so I do not believe in prayer. This does not mean that I never pray! The symbolism of an omnipotent and protecting force seems to me an inevitably attractive idea, and my own familiarity with the language of that belief offered me a ready route for calling out for help. The mountains that evoked the language of the 121st Psalm on my last night in the maternity clinic remained symbolic for me despite my occasional wish that I could be, as I was in childhood, a believer in my own importance in the grand scheme of things. But in truth, I see this wish as more whimsical than meaningful. Another thing I don't believe is the idea that "everything happens for a reason." I think that things happen, and it's up to us to create both the meaning and the purpose in all aspects of our lives.

I assume it is true to say that the impetus to be a good parent is simply part of our human makeup and that the ability to live up to that instinct is as much influenced by the kind of parenting we ourselves have received as by external resources. The lives lived by both Clive's and my parents represented a model that made it impossible for us to imagine failure as an option in parenthood. In addition, despite any misgivings I might have had about my personal strength, my own personality supported my ability to adapt to the demands of Melanie's intense fragility. My family and friends would readily describe me as the eternal optimist, and my mother's favorite story of my childhood adaptability was of a visit to my godmother in Montego Bay when I was about 6. There were many of us spending the weekend in Auntie Bertie's small house, and as the adults conversed about where we would all sleep, I was said to have exclaimed: "It's okay! I can sleep anywhere! I can fit!"

In addition to having positive internal models of parenting, we also had practical and supportive networks to turn to. Clive's father and aunt (the sister of his by-then deceased mother), as well as his then teenage nieces, Paula and Jessy, whose own mother had died in childbirth, constituted our immediate family then in Trinidad. Clive's network of siblings, who were at that time living in the United States and Toronto, were integral to our family identity and would prove to be a continuing source of support for us. My brothers, both physicians living in Toronto, were literally at the other end of the telephone line. My eldest brother, Gervais, paid a visit to see Melanie when she was just a few months old, and Philip, from the first to the last day of Melanie's life, was absolute in his involvement and support.

So we were supremely fortunate to have families from whom we knew Melanie would receive unconditional love, no matter what her needs proved to be. There was not one member of either of our families who would interpret this new member's life in negative or stigmatizing terms, not one who would hesitate to welcome her wholeheartedly into the family. I will tell here a story that all Trinidadians will understand and which I hope others unfamiliar to that culture will accept, trusting the well-intentioned, often humorous nature of Trinidad's unique mixture of racial competition and tolerance. Melanie's facial features and hair texture spoke unequivocally of her Indian heritage. On the first occasion on which we were able to take Melanie to visit her paternal grandfather, Papa—himself the classic Trinidadian *dougla*—reached out his arms to hold the newest of a dozen rainbow-colored grandchildren and, gazing at her with a huge smile, exclaimed, "Oh, Lord! I've got a Coolie grandchild at last!"

For my part, my parents were then living in Jamaica, my father increasingly incapacitated by Parkinson's disease and early-onset dementia, and my mother, herself a registered nurse, taking impeccable care of him, as she would until his death some 3 years later. It was painful to me to know that Melanie had come into our family at a point when she would not be able to benefit from her grandfather's professional experience and generous, loving spirit. My parents visited us at the time of Melanie's homecoming, and the only picture I have of Daddy with her shows him holding her tentatively, with an expression of intense anxiety and puzzlement. Meanwhile, throughout the years of Melanie's life, my mother continued to be a source of absolute support and love for Melanie, Clive, myself, and later our son Mark.

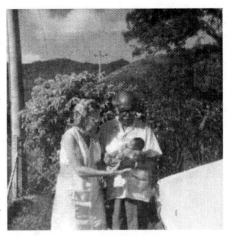

With Grandpa Val and Grandma in Trinidad

Finally, a brief summary of Clive's and my professional situations may be helpful in providing perspective for much of what will follow in my account of my experience with Melanie. After earning my bachelor's degree in English language and literature, I accepted a job as an English teacher in a middle school in Toronto and quickly found that teaching came naturally to me. By the time I left Toronto for Trinidad, I had completed my master's degree in education and had taught middle and high school as well as briefly at a community college.

In Trinidad, I was delighted to accept a job with the University of the West Indies as a lecturer in a new in-service program for high school teachers. At the time of Melanie's birth I was on maternity leave from that position. On learning of Melanie's uncertain condition, my department kindly offered me up to 6 months' leave of absence, at the end of which I could decide whether or not to return to work. Jumping ahead in my narrative, let me say here that I had no hesitation in resigning at the end of that period. We lived simply, in a modest house rented from Marlene and Eccles, Clive's sister and brother-in-law, who lived in Toronto. As Clive liked to say, the diminished income would simply mean he would have to drink rum instead of scotch! He, meanwhile, was employed as an economist in a quasi-governmental agency for industrial development—having been the manager of the agency's Toronto office before our move to Trinidad. This professional Toronto connection would prove invaluable for us as Melanie's needs became clearer.

I offer this brief personal and family history to provide some limited context for the journey on which Clive and I so unexpectedly found ourselves. Up until that time I had led a charmed life. For me, more so than for Clive, this was life's first real hurdle.

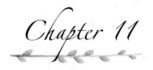

Chapter 11

"OH, GOD! NO!"

I have said much about Melanie, about Clive, and about me, but the picture would be incomplete without mention of other people. By other people, I mean everybody in my world whom I tended to classify as either supportive or unsupportive.

Melanie's nurses for the most part I considered supportive, my family and Clive's were supportive, some friends were supportive, and others were unsupportive; people on the streets were, I was sure, unsupportive; books were supportive; the dog was unsupportive, and so on!

I think that my idea of *supportive* at the time was any attitude that seemed to accept unconditionally whatever attitude *I* displayed at any given moment. To put it less facetiously, I think I probably needed a mirror or an endless series of mirrors to my very fragmented self. The situation I was in was new and frightening, and I had to come to terms with it. Coming to terms with it meant, for me, facing and grappling with numerous aspects of myself as well as with some indisputable facts. The facts had to be accepted, and my own feelings had to be understood and then either accepted or modified or, one might say, resolved.

So, for example, I felt it necessary to accept as a fact that Melanie had experienced brain damage, as the evidence seemed indisputable. As always, an essential part of acceptance for me was being able to speak the fact, to hear myself say it, and to experience the reassurance of knowing that the words were acceptable to my own ears and to the ears of my listener. One of the most unsupportive things a listener could do, therefore, was to disagree with what I was saying. Thus any well-intentioned friend or acquaintance who made the mistake of trying to reassure me by expressing disagreement about Melanie's condition would immediately fall into the category of unsupportive. To say, "But isn't the doctor jumping to conclusions?" or "Surely it's too soon to diagnose brain damage," or worst of all "Oh! There's nothing wrong with the baby, she's just weak" (or small or dysmature, or whatever), was to alienate me immediately. No doubt such comments were intended to be supportive, but I felt that they arose from what would turn out to be an unacceptable attitude to such a problem; that is, if people felt the need to deny the likelihood of Melanie's having brain damage, it was because the idea was unacceptable, perhaps even repugnant to them. They could not stand the thought and, therefore, could not stand to hear me say it. My feeling was, "If you are going to support me, you must be able to hear me say it. You must accept what I am saying."

I found that the more direct a person's acknowledgment of the problem, the more acceptable it was to me. I suspect that the only totally honest response I got from anyone was from Pat, an old friend whom I did not tell until several months after Melanie's return home. She had seen Melanie and had known that she was full of problems, but I had not told her of the diagnosis. When I did, she said, "Oh, God! No!" Here was no disguise, no modification, simply "Oh, God! No!" I was grateful for her honesty and her empathy—no rationalizing, no denial, simply the terrible mixture of disbelief and resignation that one feels in the face of fate. Most of my supportive responses were much calmer and more rational— nodding, sympathetic faces, questions for clarification, comments that emphasized the optimistic features I described, and best of all, quiet and accepting listening. These listeners provided the mirrors I needed, gave me the opportunity to give form to my fears, to somehow objectify them, and finally, to feel myself and my friend still alive and well in spite of the terrible thing that had been said.

These responses came for the most part from people of a background and education similar to mine—people perhaps, whose education and/or conditioning had given them, first of all, a faith in modern science that allowed them to accept a doctor's interpretation of the features we could all see in Melanie and, second, an attitude relatively free of superstition and traditional stigmatizing of anything strange. In addition to these attitudes, these were people of considerable social and perhaps one could say intellectual or emotional skills—that is, skills in being able to find a rational framework from which to view a terrible emotional problem—people who could say, "What on earth could've caused this?" instead of "Why should this happen to you!" or "Well, can the doctor say how serious her limitations will be?" rather than, "I don't believe it. I'm sure she'll be all right."

To these people, I could present the rational, coping side of myself, the side that was able to put my emotions into a context that made them susceptible to exploration, speculation, and resolution. To them also, I could separate what was fact from what was speculation. This was particularly important since my acceptance of the diagnosis of brain damage was qualified by my knowledge that this need not mean mental retardation since the motor functions could be impaired and the intelligence perfectly normal. The fact that I was accepting was the doctor's advice that we must expect *at least* some degree of physical disability. The speculation was: will her intelligence be normal? A supportive listener therefore had to be able to make it clear that he or she recognized this potential distinction.

I have already quoted one or two typical unsupportive responses. These stand out in my mind, and to be honest, I can think of very few other examples. Perhaps this is because there were in fact very few such responses, although at the time I thought there were many. I often used to tell Clive how impossible I found it to talk to this or that person about Melanie, and he consistently replied that he suspected that I, rather than the other person, was creating the problem. He said he thought that I anticipated an unsupportive reaction from certain people and either elicited it or read it into whatever they said. Of course I thought it unsupportive of him to make such an observation!

Some 2 years later, in a conversation with Marian, one of my most supportive friends, I gained a sudden and most revealing insight into this problem. I had long realized that the unsupportive responses tended to come, I thought, from people whom I considered relatively unsophisticated, and I had assumed that such responses were the natural properties of such people. In retrospect, I saw that both the supportive and the unsupportive responses were natural properties of myself, which I had systematically projected onto other people. My most irrational self existed, I thought, not in me but in others. *Others* would be unable to accept a flawed child. *Others* would see me as a failure as a woman. *Others* would assume that a defective brain was totally incompetent. *Others* would blind themselves to an unpleasant truth. *Others* would, after all, reject my child.

Such others, therefore, were excluded as far as possible from my situation, and with them Melanie's problems would be discussed minimally or not at all. Ironically, years later, I would find that some, whom I had largely excluded from my confidence, would be the ones to show great love and acceptance of Melanie and be, after all, very supportive.

Besides Pat's "Oh, God! No!" one other response stands out vividly in my memory. This came from a friend of my mother whom I have known all my life and who already knew of the problem at the time that she first saw Melanie. She exclaimed, "Lord! What a pretty baby!" Thank you, Aunt Des!

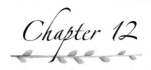

Chapter 12

THE BEARER OF BAD NEWS

I have said that I gradually came to include our pediatrician among my unsupportive public. I would like to clarify this.

First of all, I think it must be a rare mother who can succeed in not harboring some resentment toward the bearer of bad news regarding her child. It must also be the rare doctor who can carry out this unhappy task and simultaneously behave in a manner that will continue, under much pressure, to be supportive. I say *under much pressure* because most parents will probably appear to be trying to pressure the doctor into clarifying, expanding on, and perhaps even changing his original diagnosis. Indeed, all that I have read on the subject of parents' responses shows that parents are often so stunned by the first statement of the diagnosis that very little of what they are told sinks in at the time; they, therefore, keep coming back to the doctor with questions that he feels sure he has already answered. It seems only natural that he would eventually find this persistence irritating.

My own experience certainly bears this out, and in retrospect, I see many sides of the problem. First, I think the observation that the parents absorb little of what they are told on the first occasion is largely true. This is partly because they are in a state of shock and partly because their level of information and understanding of such

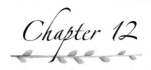 51

problems is minimal. For myself, I would say that I absorbed what fitted into my already existing framework of knowledge. For example, I had known a child with cerebral palsy and had known that his intelligence was normal. I knew also that the brain is a highly complex organ with different areas governing different functions. Had I not known this, I might well have interpreted the term *brain damage* to mean that my child's brain would not function at all. So I had a reference point for the term *brain damage.*

But there were many things I had no reference points for. It had never occurred to me, for instance, that instinctive reflexes like swallowing or sucking could be impaired by brain damage. It had never, I am sure, crossed my mind that a person might be unable to swallow. Unable to walk, or talk, or remember, but not to *swallow!* Therefore, when the doctor first suggested that the gargling in Melanie's throat might be milk that she was unable to swallow, I dismissed the suggestion. As far as I knew, milk almost automatically went down one's throat—sort of by gravity! This was something, therefore, that I had to keep asking about.

This precise lack of understanding also made me keep asking the doctor why she was drooling, which she did intermittently. All I could think of was that horrible term a *drooling idiot*, which must mean that drooling is a sign of severe mental retardation. I kept asking why she drooled, and he kept saying that it was because she was not swallowing her saliva. How simple! It could not be that simple; I mean, saliva doesn't even have to be swallowed—surely it just goes down!

The same applied to her choking. Why was she choking? After a while, I sensed irritation in the doctor's responses, which he (quite reasonably) started to preface with "As I told you before . . . ."

So I think that one of the main reasons for unsatisfactory communication between the doctor and the parents is the gap in their respective prior knowledge and experience. This of course is reinforced by the fact that the new knowledge is largely repugnant to the parent, and he or she consequently becomes a very slow learner.

This brings me to the second point: the conflict between wanting to know and not wanting to know. I certainly wanted to know, but I wanted to know only what I was ready to accept. Yet I insisted on asking.

And so the question of our doctor's continuing assessment of Melanie's progress became a terrible problem for me. The sum of it was that his opinion of her performance and possible potential kept going down.

As I have said, when he gave me his diagnosis 3 or 4 weeks after her birth, he indicated some optimism based on the fact that she was trying to lift her head when lying on her stomach. Also, her head circumference had grown at a reasonably promising rate.

Toward the end of November, my hopes and general morale were significantly lifted by a visit from my oldest brother, Gervais, who is a physician. He came from Toronto to see his new niece and to offer moral support and hopefully some clarification of the medical interpretation of her condition.

He spent an evening with our pediatrician, and his sharing with us of that interview was quite encouraging. He impressed upon us, as had our very supportive family doctor, Dr. Roache, the tremendous complexity of the brain and the infinite possibilities regarding types of brain damage.

In particular, the pediatrician had stressed to Gervais the noticeable disparity between Melanie's being unable to perform the most primitive of functions such as swallowing and sucking and yet being able to lift her head up from prone lying at the age of 10 weeks. So I knew that at that time, Dr. McDowall was still focusing on the strengths Melanie was demonstrating.

At about 3 months, however, he observed that the rate of head growth had slowed considerably and that this was not a good sign. By 4 months, Melanie was trying to hold up her head when held at my shoulder, and this he said was good, but this was counteracted by her lack of development in other areas. He had what I called his list of 10 questions that he asked every time we went (Clive always went with me), and to which we constantly had to answer *no*. His questions centered on whether she was trying to follow a moving object (she always failed his flashlight test for this), or turning her head toward a sound or voice, or trying to reach for an object, or to us most important of all, smiling.

I pressed him for an interpretation of these facts. By then, I had read of the general classification of mental retardation on a scale from profound to mild, and soon after she was 4 months old, I put the question to him: She was not blind, apparently, so why was she not responding? I remember his words vividly. "It is not a matter of vision, it is a matter of interpretation."

So I pressed, "She can see, but does not understand what she can see. What does this mean?" He replied that there must be some degree of mental retardation although he pointed out that it was early to say how great this disability might be. I insisted that he suggest the level at which he thought she was functioning—where would he classify her at this point in time? He said probably in the range of moderate retardation—not mild, since her lack of responsiveness was still so marked, and not severe, since she was showing signs of developing some head control.

I was shaking as we left his office, and by the time we got to the car, my control was totally gone. I was hurt, angry, disappointed, resentful, disbelieving, and believing—everything at once. A mixture of belief and disbelief was, I think, one of the main features of my response. On the one hand, the doctor's explanation of Melanie's lack of response seemed perfectly reasonable. Like him, I felt sure she was seeing, for when I would come within her line of vision, her gaze seemed so intent that it was hard to doubt her sight, but she never seemed to try to follow what she had seen, and sometimes she would even seem to be deliberately turning away from whatever the stimulus was. So it was not hard to assume that this lack of response must arise from lack of motivation or interest or understanding, whichever is the main feature of mental deficiency.

Yet the intensity of gaze that I just described made it difficult to believe that there was no understanding. When Melanie looked at a person, her expression seemed both intentional and intelligent. Of course, it probably seemed especially so to me, but there were several people who described her as seeming alert and attentive.

Quite apart from any rationalizing about or observing of Melanie, I simply was not ready to think of the possibility of her having intellectual delays. The word *retarded* was in fact a word I felt I would probably never be able to use in relation to Melanie; she might have brain damage or cerebral palsy or anything but mental retardation.

I had known only a few people with children with intellectual disabilities, and my main response had always been one of intense pity. The worst aspect of the situation seemed to me to be the plight of the parents, who I assumed would forever have to carry the burden of a dependent person and to worry about what would happen to this child when they were gone. To know that your child would never grow up seemed an impossible burden to bear.

Not long before Melanie's birth, I had heard some friends referring to a couple they knew whose child had intellectual disabilities and saying that the mother, who used to be quite attractive, now looked worn and plain. I had thought to myself that this must surely be inevitable in such a situation. Who could survive such a catastrophe even physically intact?

So while on one level I believed the doctor, on another I did not and found it impossible to discuss this assessment with anyone but Clive. Clive's response was, "It's too early to tell, let's wait and see." And for once, I really tried to follow this advice.

I watched Melanie like a hawk. If there was going to be any sign of response, I would see it. By 5 months, Melanie was able to flip onto her back by pushing up on her hands and appearing to lose her balance. Whether or not this move was voluntary, I couldn't tell, but she did voluntarily try to roll from her back onto her stomach and had actually been successful on a few occasions. Her head control continued to improve although her head movements, like all her movements, had a stiffness about them that made them seem somewhat unnatural. Clive used to say she looked like a little lizard, lying on her tummy with her head sticking up stiff and straight and turning from side to side.

I was by now convinced that she could not move her eyes and was beginning to develop a theory that the control center for the eyes must be damaged, but I had no support for such an idea. The other part of Melanie that moved very little was her face; her features were relatively immobile. The frown of her early months was by now almost gone, but there was very little expression in its place. Her face did not register any of the normal range of expressions such as surprise, anger, pleasure, or puzzlement, but what baffled me was that her *body* did.

As I have said before, she would respond to sounds by somehow changing her level of activity or by crying or stopping a cry. Somewhere in her 6th month, it occurred to me to really test her vision by seeing if the sight of me would elicit such a response. It did!

I put her in her little prop-up chair on the sofa in the living room, left the room, and some minutes later stepped silently into the doorway between the kitchen and the living room directly in her line of vision. She responded immediately with a clear startle, a sudden jerk of arms and legs, and a movement of the head. For weeks, I repeated this little experiment day after day, and day after day I received the same response, and occasionally if I had been out of the room longer than usual, a cry.

I was greatly encouraged; Melanie was definitely seeing, but more important, she was responding. Surely, she must also be interpreting. What else would account for an immediate and consistent physical response to my appearing? Although her expression changed little, surely her body was registering an emotional response of some sort. What could have made the experiment more meaningful, I now see, would have been to try the same test with another person and see if there was a difference in response. But in any case, whether or not she was in fact recognizing *me* in particular, she was seeing and responding.

But there were no smiles, no reaching out for the world. And when she was close to 6 months, the doctor responded to my continued insistent questioning with the opinion that her level of mental retardation now seemed to be pretty severe.

In the car afterwards, Clive, still willing to hold the doctor's opinion in abeyance for a while, could not help pointing out that, after pressing the doctor for his opinion, I was now angry because I did not like his opinion.

Clive was right.

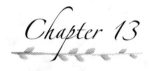

NESTARGEL

There were two things that carried me through those months: one was the incredible demand of caring for Melanie, and the other was my planned trip to Canada. I will speak of each in turn.

Melanie's homecoming on November 25, 1975, marked the beginning of a year and a half of uninterrupted anxiety over her feeding. For the first 2 months or so, the problem seemed to be in a period of transition between her learning to swallow and her learning to vomit when the swallowing failed. I kept records of every feeding—the amount taken, the efficiency of her swallowing, and an estimate of the amount regurgitated. The notes show three patterns in her feeding. Sometimes she would vomit both during and after the feeding, at which times the difficulty in swallowing was usually evident. Sometimes she would appear to have swallowed perfectly throughout the feeding and would then spend anywhere from 15 minutes to 2 hours bringing it up. And at other times, perhaps once a day or maybe only once in a few days, she would swallow and retain the whole feeding. The second pattern was perhaps the hardest to understand. If the vomiting was related to inefficient swallowing, what was the cause of the excessive vomiting after an apparently successful feeding?

Melanie's vomiting was not the dramatic projectile vomiting in which the food shoots out and lands some feet away; it was a gentle spilling out of anything from 1 to 1½ ounces at a time. Dr. McDowall speculated that the cause was a weak sphincter muscle at the entrance to the stomach and recommended that Melanie be propped upright after every feeding, the idea being that the force of gravity would help to keep the food down. This had no effect whatever; in fact, a pattern emerged in which her best feeding was her evening bedtime feeding, after which she was put directly to lie down and fall asleep quickly.

We tried many approaches: giving smaller, more frequent feedings; larger, less frequent feedings; thicker feedings, thinner feedings, slower feedings, and faster feedings. We tried getting her to sleep right after every feeding, but this only worked at bedtime. The problem seemed totally beyond our control.

There was a tendency for her to retain and to swallow more easily a feeding that had been thickened with cereal or potato or banana, and so for a while I concentrated on this. These feedings stayed down quite well for a couple of weeks, but this soon became less consistent.

Somewhere in early April, our pediatrician suggested a food-thickening agent called Nestargel. We had heard of it before from a friend who had used it with her baby, but we had thought its starchy consistency would have made it too difficult for Melanie to swallow. I managed to obtain a bottle of this powder, the last bottle the agents had, and started trying it with Melanie.

The swallowing turned out to be no problem, and I subsequently realized that, in fact, heavy substances were much easier for Melanie to swallow than light ones.

Within a day or two, I felt that the miracle had finally happened. We had found the answer to Melanie's vomiting! The Nestargel was working like a charm—apparently, its sheer weight kept the food down, for Melanie was vomiting only minimally. I gradually increased the use of the Nestargel until I was including it in every feeding, and for about a month its success was quite consistent. Melanie's rate of weight gain increased dramatically. Looking over my notes, I saw a clear pattern of improvement. It had taken her from March 4 until April 8, over a month, to gain 4 ounces (from 7 pounds to 7 pounds and 4 ounces). I started the Nestargel on April 7. She gained 4 ounces in the following week, 4 the next week, and 7 in the following two weeks, so that in the first month using the Nestargel, her weight jumped from 7 pounds 6 ounces to 8 pounds 3 ounces on May 6. One week after that, on May 13, she weighed 8 pounds and 10 ounces, having finally doubled her birth weight.

Melanie was at that point almost 8 months old, and she weighed what many babies weigh at birth, but I was delighted with the big jump in her weight, and to me, she was actually beginning to look chubby in the cheeks!

She was awake pretty well all day, taking perhaps two 10-minute catnaps and fretting much of the time in between. Her nights were not too bad, however, as she usually woke just once between her 9:00–10:00 p.m. bedtime and her 6:00–7:00 a.m. rising. The gargling response of her early months had by then disappeared, although she would often be very uncomfortable for a long time after a feeding, making little clicking noises in her throat and fretting and arching her neck and back.

She still had frequent choking spasms in which she suddenly began to gasp and choke; it had taken me months to realize that I could get her out of them quite easily by turning her on her side and patting her back to enable the saliva or food to drain out. Most times, it did appear to be her saliva that for some reason she simply could not swallow at that moment. I had learned to handle these spasms, but not without fear.

I think it is true to say that the only consistent enjoyment I had of Melanie was at her bedtime, which had become quite predictably her best feeding, after which she was always peaceful and sleepy. I would sing her my Sweet Bird song and pat her back. She would go off to sleep, and I would feel, for a few moments, like a normal mother.

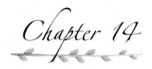

THE SPIRAL STAIRCASE

Whatever release was denied me in caring for Melanie, I made up for in my imagination. My few spare moments became signals to escape into fantasies of my forthcoming trip to Toronto.

It had been only 3 years since Clive and I had moved to Trinidad. Consequently, we both identified quite strongly with Canada, and we both had family still living there as well as close friends and many contacts of different kinds. Most people in a developing country who find themselves with a baby with problems like Melanie's will consider the possibility of going to a developed country for advice and/or medical help. We were fortunate in having the kind of network that made this easy for us, and we had started talking about the trip soon after we knew of Melanie's problem.

By the time she was 4 months old, I had written to the Ontario Crippled Children's Center (OCCC) for advice as to when to bring her for an assessment and had received an encouraging reply. Our main plan was to go to that institution as soon as the northern climate started becoming more hospitable. We would go in the spring, we decided, and set the date for the middle of May.

Sometime in March, I heard from my mother that a childhood friend of mine, who was also my mother's goddaughter, was now a doctor living in New York and studying to be a *physiatrist*. This was a new term to me, but I gathered that her work involved the physical rehabilitative treatment of children whose movements have been negatively affected by conditions such as cerebral palsy. In great excitement, I wrote off to my friend Pat, and in the next 2 months we communicated both by letter and by phone. Pat's main point was that the form of therapy that she would recommend (neurodevelopmental therapy, as it was called, though I later came to know it by the simpler term Bobath therapy, named after its originator, Vera Bobath) should be started as early as possible with any baby who has cerebral palsy. She gave me great encouragement with her letters, phone calls, and the promise of an appointment for assessment at her hospital, Blythedale Hospital in New York State.

With these two appointments in view, I had much to look forward to. It was not that I expected these visits to provide any miracle cure for Melanie; I tend to be skeptical on the subject of miracles at the best of times, and certainly in this case I knew that medicine could not cure brain damage. But I felt sure that the visit would offer me an educated opinion on Melanie as well as practical guidance in handling her and, I hoped, some emotional support. I believe, in fact, that the latter was my greatest objective.

As the months passed, Toronto became my mecca. I became more and more nostalgic for the city in which I had spent all my adult life, for I had left home at 18 to go to university there. I had grown into adulthood in Toronto and had made all my first adult decisions there. My adult friendships had been formed there, and my advanced education and professional training and experience were all gained there.

Going to Toronto at this time of crisis, then, would be going home. I would have my brothers, my sisters-in-law, three dear women friends, and knowledgeable and experienced doctors and therapists. I could think of little else.

The importance of this feeling expressed itself most forcefully in a dream that I recorded on April 6, whose powerful images spoke vividly of the tremendous hopes on which my trip hinged, and of course the fear of failure that is implicit in every hope. My notes read:

A dream of a spiral staircase, at the side of a large building like Centennial College or Newtonbrook High, schools in which I had taught in Toronto. In the midst of some function, I leave through a side door and go running down a long, winding, spiraling staircase made of wrought iron or steel with open sides. It is outdoors, at night, and the staircase seems set against a brilliant night sky, pitch black with very bright stars standing out in contrast to the blackness. As I descend, it becomes evident that there is a large crowd, apparently attending the same function, and they stand all along the staircase. Finally I realize that either the staircase ends in a cul-de-sac, or else the door at the end is locked. I am confused and surprised, as this is not how it used to be. I realize that *they,* possibly the administration of the institution, have blocked off the route, perhaps for purposes of this function. By this time, I am in the midst of a large crowd, and since there is no exit, I realize I must make my way back up. I am very upset and bothered by this. As I start back, I meet my cousin, Maggie, coming toward me. As we begin to talk the dream fades.

The next day, as the associations started flooding in, I saw that the staircase, the central image of the dream, was a composite of many images. It was reminiscent of the stairs at Piarco Airport in Trinidad where people stand peering through the windows below for a glimpse of the arriving passengers. A wrought-iron staircase, its open sides, suggested at once the precarious promise of an outdoor fire escape as well as the confinement of burglar-proofed windows, and for me, the echo of the *decorative grilles,* a phrase familiar to me from Louise Bogan's "Evening in the Sanitarium," a poem about a mental asylum. Only the day before, I had been aware of the total impossibility of my beautiful Little Bird ever being caged within the confines of an institution.

Also, on the previous day, a friend, returning from Toronto, had spoken of a students' residence in which the presence of iron grilles, on the windows had indicated that the city was no longer as safe as it used to be.

And so, on one level, the staircase definitely represented Toronto and my view of it as a fire escape—an escape through a well-known old route. This route is very attractive and open as the stairs shine their hope against the blackness of the night sky. At first I am moving quickly, easily, very sure-footed, and light on my feet, but I slow down as the crowd thickens and doubt about the exit develops. So this could be interpreted as a warning that the old route has changed, the exit is blocked, and this route does not provide an escape.

But of course, on a wider level, the dream says that there is no escape from Melanie's problems and that even the most attractive-looking escape has negative connotations, such as the iron grillework, so attractive yet so reminiscent of burglar proofing, and the poem about the mental institution. Institutionalizing Melanie would not provide an escape, nor would insanity nor neurosis nor crowds of friends or strangers.

I cannot use the past as an escape, cannot recapture the light-footedness, the sure-footedness of those years. Neither can I escape through crowds of people, for their exit is also blocked, and they appear to be using the staircase as a viewing point for the function. If these are the people who wait for me, they are not looking in my direction and are using the cul-de-sac for some other purpose. To them, it is a viewing gallery, to me, a cul-de-sac.

Overall, I could see that the dream represented my disappointment regarding Melanie. I had started the pregnancy joyfully, confident, full of expectations, sure that I knew the way. Then came the shock of finding myself on an unexpected route, a route from which there was no exit. Now I was trapped and must make my way back to the starting point—a new beginning.

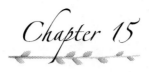

Chapter 15

SMILING

In the month before we were due to leave for Toronto, Melanie started smiling. She was 7 months old, and the moment we had awaited for many months was every bit as wonderful and rewarding as we could ever have imagined! The moment was unquestionably distinct, because unlike normal babies Melanie had not displayed any of the little smirks, half-smiles, and generally questionable movements of the mouth that parents fondly interpret as smiles. I had seen her smile in her sleep once or twice, but her waking expression had continued to be steadily somber.

So there was no doubt about her first smile: one day Clive whistled at her (for about the millionth time) and she smiled. I had not seen it, and when he told me, I was incredulous. That night, he whistled again, and this time, I was there. It was a beautiful one-sided smile, clear and distinct, and I felt I would die of gratitude!

From then on, Clive whistled as if his life depended on it. The smiles were not frequent, but they were consistently distinct and came only in response to Clive's whistles—no other whistle, no other stimulus would do. But this was more than enough for me—Melanie was smiling, and her smile was beautiful and meaningful.

So with one or two dozen smiles under our belts, Melanie and I left for Toronto on May 16. We were met by Jo, my brother Philip's wife, whose tearful greeting came as spontaneously as

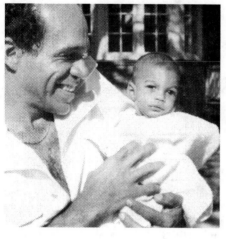

Melanie at 7 months with Uncle Philip in Toronto

mine—we had each been through our separate traumas in the previous year.

After my initial correspondence with OCCC, Philip had acted as the referring doctor for us and had made the assessment appointment. After a joyful yet tearful greeting, exclamations over Melanie's beauty, and Philip's observation that her spasticity didn't seem too bad to him, my big question was, when was the assessment? He had made it for the 18th, only a few days away. This was fine with me as I still wasn't sure how long we'd be staying and was anxious to get on with it.

Melanie and I were staying with my friend Georgia, who had visited with us in March and so already knew the Sweet Bird. It felt so wonderful to be back in the fold, as it were, back in an environment full of friends and family with whom I had shared other important periods in my life, long-standing relationships whose solidity I trusted because of years of experience. My relationships in Trinidad were wonderful but much newer and, therefore, up to that time, less sure. My parents had stayed with us for 2 months after Melanie's homecoming, and despite my father's ill health, their presence had made me realize how much I needed the support of really committed relationships during that period of crisis.

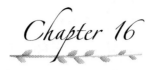

INITIAL ASSESSMENTS

Our appointment at the OCCC was set for May 18th at 12:30 p.m. Georgia dropped us there, and within minutes we were met by a young woman who took us to sit in the waiting lounge. She introduced herself as Sally Speers and explained that she would be our guide for the afternoon. She was a pleasant and intelligent young woman, herself affected by cerebral palsy. Her gait and speech clearly indicated this condition, and my initial reaction was to feel sympathetic toward her. I felt myself instinctively being gentle in my conversation with her as if she would naturally need my protection.

It didn't take long before I realized how inappropriate this reaction was. Surely in this situation I was the vulnerable one! I was the one who stood shaking behind a calm exterior, feeling as though my whole life lay helplessly in the hands of these people. Sally Speers had coped well with her own problem and was now there to help me with mine.

I was also interviewed by a young woman from admissions, whose job it was simply to record factual information of the type that every institution requires for its files. She performed this task with gentleness and grace, and I felt I was among friends. It was apparent that this would not be like the assessments I had read of in mothers' reports, with cold–fish–like interviews and endless red tape.

Soon Dr. Wilmington appeared. I had been prepared for the fact that he was in a wheelchair as I had heard this by the grapevine, but I was not prepared for the kindness of his face and the friendly gentleness of his manner. As he led me down the hall, he chatted about Melanie's size, observing that she was probably the smallest and among the youngest babies to be assessed at the center. By the time we got to the CP Unit, where the assessment would be conducted, I knew that I was going to be made to feel as comfortable as possible. The therapists, an occupational therapist and a physical therapist, fit in with the pattern. They were cheerful and friendly, and the whole approach was relaxed and informal.

I cannot describe the assessment in any great detail. Like the first conversation with our pediatrician, of which I could remember only certain features against a hazy background, this assessment remains in my memory like an impressionist painting upon which a student of realism has superimposed six or seven contrasting strokes. I think the best I can do is to describe these strokes.

One feature that remains vividly with me was the therapists' tone of supportiveness in handling Melanie. The whole process was laced with positive reinforcement and an affectionate manner. Every time they said, "Good girl, Melanie," I found myself thinking, *God! They are actually on her side!* Why I should have expected them to be against her, I don't know.

I remember them asking me if she knew my voice; I called to her, "Hello, Sweet Bird," and was grateful when she responded by freezing in her activity and looking attentive, although she did not turn to look at me. I was even more grateful when they agreed that she certainly did know my voice.

Of the doctor's examination of her, I remember only that he could not get her mouth open. I remember him saying after his examination was complete that he was "not convinced of the spasticity." He was referring to our pediatrician's report in which he diagnosed her as having spastic-type cerebral palsy. I did not at the moment understand what the OCCC doctor meant by this comment. I remember that a speech therapist and a psychologist also participated and recall describing the feeding problem to the speech therapist.

After this phase of the assessment was over, the doctor told me that he would send Melanie on to be seen by their consultant neurologist and ophthalmologist.

The latter referral related to the fact that this doctor expressed grave doubts about her vision. He was getting practically no response to his tests on this area and asked me whether I thought she could see. My brother, Philip, had expressed the same doubts, but in both cases, I replied that I was sure she had vision. I knew for sure that she responded to the sight of me, for I had, as I described earlier, tested this over and over. However, I was glad for the referral. We proceeded directly to the neurologist and then to the ophthalmologist.

Of the whole afternoon's proceedings, it was only my conversation with the neurologist that caused me any feeling of unhappiness. I was asking his opinion about Melanie's vision and generally unresponsive facial expression, to which he replied that while she might be seeing, it was probably just that she "couldn't care less" about what she saw. This colloquial phrasing and his generally offhand manner offended me deeply. To say, as our pediatrician at home had, that she might not be able to *interpret* what she saw was somehow far more acceptable, even though it meant the same thing.

In any case, the ophthalmologist confirmed that there was nothing wrong with the structure of her eyes but was reluctant to offer an interpretation, saying that she was still very young and should be studied and observed again within a year.

After some hours of meeting with various members of this professional team, it was time for a summary meeting conducted by Dr. Wilmington and the two therapists.

Overall, there were two main points that stayed in my mind—first, that there was some doubt about the nature of Melanie's cerebral palsy. The neurologist had been quite sure that she demonstrated features of athetoid cerebral palsy, which include fluctuating muscle tone and a tendency to too much, rather than too little, movement. Dr. Wilmington, on the other hand, doubted this diagnosis yet was not convinced that she was spastic either, this latter type meaning increased muscle tone resulting in the evident tightness of the limbs.

It seemed to me that if this doctor doubted that she was either athetoid or spastic, then it probably meant that he did not think she had cerebral palsy at all. I knew enough to understand that if a motor disability was ruled out, the remaining diagnosis would probably be severe mental retardation. In other words, if the damage was to areas of the brain that affect muscle tone and movement, then that could explain delayed development in many areas; but if the known symptoms of motor impairment were not there, then the cause of delay would be a more generalized, low-functioning intelligence.

Yet Dr. Wilmington would not say that. He said, rather, and this was the second point that stayed with me, that she was too young yet for him to make any valid judgment about the extent of her *developmental delay* (a new term for me, which I took to be a euphemism for mental retardation) and that he would recommend waiting until she was at least 2 and certainly until she was over her severe feeding problems.

Despite the uncertainty of this kind of diagnosis, the wait-and-see approach was quite acceptable to me, and I felt considerable relief at the end of the interview. It was clear that doors had been opened for study of Melanie's condition and that they would remain open for our use. In fact, the interview ended with the setting of an appointment for that Friday, only 3 days away, in which the therapists would work with my Sweet Bird and me with a view to teaching me how best to help her. This assessment then was not to be an end in itself but rather a beginning.

It was, in fact, the beginning of what would turn out to be a long and varied relationship with the Ontario Crippled Children's Center.

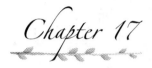

SEEING

So! We were in Toronto and had made a new start. The plan was that Melanie and I were to be at Georgia's for 3 weeks, at which time Clive would be joining us for at least a 3-week holiday or, at best, a temporary transfer to Trinidad and Tobago's Industrial Development Corporation (IDC) office in Toronto. Although Clive had been working quietly on this possibility, it just seemed too wonderful to be anything but a dream, so I had geared myself to being in Toronto for about 6 weeks.

The first 3 weeks at Georgia's rushed by with a rapid flow of events for Melanie and me. First, of course, we had to establish our accustomed feeding routines with a comfortable chair in the living room and a footrest to prop my legs on, since Melanie still sat on my lap, back propped against my knees, for feeding. This posture ensured that her head was firmly placed, and I could concentrate on her face and her sounds.

The point here was the urgent need to concentrate on Melanie at all times during her feeding. Although she now swallowed fairly well, her tendency to choke suddenly on the food was still a matter of concern. Worse, although her vomiting had decreased with the Nestargel, she seemed now to be developing more of a tendency to what the therapists described as a nasal reflux, wherein the liquid being vomited flowed up and out through the nose as much, or more than, as through her mouth. Every mother knows the fears that rise at the sight of this happening to her child.

By this time, I was so totally attuned to Melanie's sounds that I could tell from the next room when she was about to vomit or from her face and the pace of her breathing when she had not swallowed properly or was in any discomfort whatever. Indeed, it is true to say that I breathed with Melanie through her feedings, involuntarily holding my breath until hers was released and taking a little gasp along with her when the swallowing process had taken so long that she had to gasp as she came up for air.

Our therapy session on Friday, May 21st, turned out to be the first of many opportunities. The OCCC staff were very concerned that I learn as much as possible before returning to Trinidad and scheduled regular sessions in which I learned many important principles of handling Melanie—positioning exercises for improving head control and developing sitting balance and methods of encouraging her to use her hands in play, which so far she was not doing at all.

But the turning point in terms of assessment of Melanie came on Friday, June 4th. The OCCC had referred us to the neonatology department of Toronto's famous Hospital for Sick Children, and on this day, Melanie, who had just passed 8 months of age and weighed the great sum of 9 pounds and 2 ounces, was introduced to a doctor whose observations and continuing interest were to prove the most important and far-reaching as far as real understanding of her condition was concerned.

Dr. Karen Pape of the Sick Kids' Neonatology Department was young and keen. The spontaneity and freshness of her approach turned my mind around and taught me probably more than I will ever learn again about how to look at a child as the child is, without bias and preconceived notions.

I cannot say how long we stayed in Dr. Pape's office or how the interview began or ended. I can say only that it seemed hours that

I sat watching her talk and play with Melanie, trying to stimulate her interest with a number of toys. The toy she persisted with longest was a bristly, bright green rubber caterpillar that squeaked when pressed. I was truly amazed at Dr. Pape's persistence, especially since Melanie seemed to me the least interested in this particular toy. I could see that she was responding with a lot of movement and sound, but it did appear that she spent more of her time turning away from this noisy, psychedelic creature than looking at it. But this doctor was obviously fascinated with Melanie's behavior, and I sat on the edge of my chair wondering what it was all about. Finally, Dr. Pape turned to me and began asking what I observed about Melanie's eyes.

In a previous chapter, I have explained my own observations on this. I was quite convinced that up to that time, I had never seen Melanie move her eyes but rather noticed that when she moved her head, the eyeballs would end up in the corner opposite to the direction she had turned.

I described these observations to her, and she agreed that she noticed the same thing. What Dr. Pape did that I had never done was to carry that observation to its logical conclusion. Since Melanie could apparently not shift her eyes to follow a moving object, what she was doing was turning her head *away* from an object so as to allow the eyes to slide into the opposite corner. In doing this, she was then looking at the object out of the corner of her eyes!

If an object was presented to her directly in the midline of her vision, she could attend, looking straight ahead at it. But if the object was then moved, say to the left, instead of moving her eyes to the left or moving her head toward the left and having to adjust the eyes as she did so, Melanie was trying to compensate for the lack of eye control by turning her head to the right, *away* from the object, thus causing her eyes to find themselves in the left corner!

As she explained this, Dr. Pape had Melanie demonstrate the process with the green caterpillar. I watched in amazement and realized that she was right; I could hardly believe that, with all my close observation, I had never noticed this.

Dr. Pape went on to try to put this aspect of Melanie's development into the context of overall brain structure and function. This was new ground for me. She described the brain in terms of three basic sections—the cerebral cortex, or frontal area; the cerebellum in the middle; and the brain stem at the base of the brain. The cortex, she explained, is known to have as its main function intelligence and some control of gross motor (large muscle) development. The cerebellum, whose functions are not yet well understood, is known to have much control over muscle coordination, fine motor (small muscle) control, and eye–hand coordination; that is, getting the eyes and hands to work together in order to manipulate materials. The brain stem is responsible for many reflexes such as swallowing, sucking, blinking of the eyes, and so on. The latter, of course, were the functions that we had known to be impaired from the time of Melanie's birth. Dr. Pape agreed with our pediatrician in Trinidad that this was certainly indicative of brain-stem damage. Beyond that certainty she felt everything was speculation at that stage. She would have to be very tentative in expressing her own speculations but shared them with me anyhow.

I did not realize then, partly through ignorance and partly through a fear of hoping for too much, how significant Dr. Pape's speculations would be in the evolution of a meaningful diagnosis of Melanie's condition. But I clung to them as the only glimmer of real hope that had so far been offered.

Melanie, she said, gave her the impression of someone with severe cerebellar damage, who may or may very well *not* have suffered damage to the cerebral cortex. In other words, it could be possible that while the brain stem and cerebellum might be damaged, resulting in impaired reflexes, poor coordination of hands, eyes, and possibly even facial movement, the cortex, with its control over intelligence and large muscle movement, could be intact. However, Dr. Pape pointed out that even if that were the case, gross damage to the lower sections could interfere with the transmission of information to the cortex and also with the person's ability to express what they know.

Of course I had known that the term *cerebral palsy* was based on this sort of condition, but having the structural aspects of it explained to me really helped to clarify the implications. For example, it was true that Melanie had continued to make slow but steady progress in gross motor development—trying to lift her head up quite early. I have pictures of her at 4 months with head quite erect, rolling over from tummy to back by 5 months, and by 7 months, she could also turn from back to stomach. This was observed on the Crippled Children's Center report when she was 8 months old. Yet up to that time she did not use her hands at all, and her eye control was very inefficient and abnormal.

Dr. Pape did not want to give me any unsubstantiated hopes but made it clear that she felt that while Melanie would certainly be described as having cerebral palsy, it was far too early to make any judgments about her intellectual development given the seriousness of her motor impairment. Even if her instinctive feeling about Melanie were correct and her intelligence really was quite intact, it would remain to be seen whether the cerebral cortex would be able to develop its potential given the severe limitations of the other parts of the brain.

Dr. Pape concluded on a hopeful note: As far as she was concerned, the door was open to further interpretation and discovery of Melanie's potential. "Keep an open mind," she emphasized, "and always be on the lookout for indicators of developing intelligence." Years later, Dr. Pape would test her theory with fascinating results.

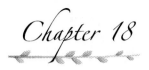

INTERPRETING

We had come to Toronto for assessment of Melanie, and assessment was the order of the day. We were due at Blythedale Hospital in New York on June 10, and to my great relief Clive would be coming in time to accompany us. By the time Clive arrived on Saturday, June 6th, Melanie and I were well ensconced in Georgia's massive bedroom, which she had vacated for us, and enjoying a continuous flow of friends and family offering their support.

My anxious dream of Toronto had been partly wrong after all. While my old home could not provide an escape, it certainly did provide support, and in massive doses. The people on the waving gallery of my dream *were* friends and were there to meet me and Melanie.

Clive's sisters, my brothers, my friends Helen and Cathy, and the warm, cushioning atmosphere of Georgia's home provided us with the cocoon we needed for safety and personal regeneration. Against this background, Georgia and Philip were the pillars on which Melanie and I leaned day in day out. Simply put, I would say that Georgia took care of me, and Philip took care of his beautiful little niece. I depended on Philip to share every day's concern regarding Melanie—the amount she had vomited, the slight fever she was running, the delivery of the dietary supplement that I had been advised to put into her milk, and innumerable other details to which he listened with infinite patience and interest.

So by the time Clive arrived, we were settled comfortably. When he walked in, Melanie was lying in the playpen. He went up to her and whistled; she gave her biggest smile ever and made a little noise that we were beginning to recognize as her squeal of delight! She certainly knew her daddy.

Clive brought good news that it seemed his temporary transfer to Toronto might really be coming through and might be for as long as 6 months. I was delighted, but we still had to wait for confirmation of this plan.

Meanwhile, it was on with the assessments. Having Clive's company for the New York trip was a great comfort to me and, I think, to Melanie. This trip also had a very welcoming aspect since we were staying at the home of Clive's brother and his family, and the assessment had been arranged by my childhood friend Pat, now a doctor at the hospital.

Over the years, I have come to think that women make more receptive doctors than men, perhaps because of a willingness to trust their instincts and to combine information so gained with information gleaned from books. While this may very well be no more than a piece of female chauvinism on my part, I freely confess that by the time we were finished at Blythedale, I was convinced of the truth of my theory.

Dr. Challenor, a physiatrist working mainly with children with brain damage, coordinated this assessment. Like Dr. Pape, she seemed able to approach Melanie unencumbered by any particular preconceptions but absolutely open to discovering whatever there was to know about the individual person that was Melanie.

Really, I think the crucial point was that these two doctors were more concerned with what Melanie *did* than with what she did *not* do. For example, Dr. Challenor took particular note of Melanie's sounds and greatly surprised me by observing that Melanie was making deliberate attempts to get my attention by using a slightly different tone, which she described as a questioning inflection. She paid great attention to these details and, in her report, wrote, "Melanie's variety of inflections is considerable, and definitely seems to be used in response to the environment. She has a clear but soft questioning inflection, which she uses to attract her mother's attention."

What an amazingly different interpretation from our pediatrician at home, who had once asked, "Is she still making that noise?" and felt that she was repeating the noise merely because she had learned how to do it, not because it had any meaning; or to the doctor at the Ontario Center, whose report commented, "She was making continuous noises, but these were quite irrelevant."

To the contrary, Dr. Challenor and Dr. Pape had both observed what Melanie *was* doing with her eyes rather than what she was *not* doing, such as *not* following a light or *not* blinking when a hand was waved in front of her eyes. Dr. Challenor confirmed that it was easier for Melanie to attend to an object presented when her eyes were at the midline and that if her eyes happened to be directed to the side, she could not voluntarily bring them back to the middle. She further observed that Melanie was consistently trying to turn her head to follow a person who had appeared in the midline of her vision.

Overall, the diagnosis of Dr. Challenor's team was that Melanie's condition was certainly cerebral palsy, possibly of the athetoid type, with delayed general development. Her report summarized this in the following way:

The combination of neuromuscular difficulties have resulted in marked developmental delays, although it

is difficult to give any meaningful estimate of probable
intellectual capacity on the basis of one examination of
a child with such motor problems within the first years
of life.

Once more then, the advice was that we would have to work
with Melanie and wait to see what she would reveal of herself
over the years.

We had had three assessments of Melanie in the 4 weeks
since leaving Trinidad, and at the time, I was very unsure of what
had really been achieved. Overall, the opinions given had left me
with more hope than I had been offered at home in that all were
saying that it was too soon to make any reliable judgment about
Melanie's potential. No prognosis at present was better than a
bad prognosis! In addition, two of the assessments had revealed
to me details of Melanie's behavior that I, who had known every
inch of this little person, had never realized. However, this report
of Melanie's early assessments would be incomplete without some
attempt to put them into perspective over time.

I have described the kindness and warmth with which
Melanie and I were received at all three centers, the OCCC, the
Hospital for Sick Children, and Blythedale Hospital. All were
attempting to give a fair and humane assessment of this little girl
with severe disabilities. In retrospect, however, I cannot help
seeing how much more perceptive and observant were the latter
two. Somehow, Dr. Pape and Dr. Challenor were able to interpret
behaviors that were so far from the norm as to be generally
unrecognizable to the average eye, even to the eye of a mother
better tuned to the child than anyone and more anxious than
anyone to see the positive. Melanie's eye movements and
vocalizing were so different from the typical appearance and
babbling activities of the average child that they seemed to
indicate practically no vision and meaningless sound. After all,

Melanie did not even move her lips when she vocalized—they were all throat sounds.

It was the absence of the typical appearances that struck the OCCC team and our doctor at home, while it was the presence of atypical behaviors that provided the focus for the attention of Dr. Pape and Dr. Challenor. From my own retrospective view, through the years of experience with Melanie that followed, I can say with certainty that the perceptions of these marvelous women were far closer to revealing truths about Melanie than were any others.

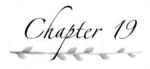

Chapter 19

SWALLOWING

By mid-June the wonderful news had been confirmed that Clive would be taking up work at the Toronto office of Trinidad's IDC. The posting was to be for about 6 months and would not be difficult for Clive since he had worked in this office before we had left Toronto between 1971 and 1973.

I have spoken before of my own inclination to be optimistic about life—a feeling of confidence in the likelihood that things will work out in the end. Clive's posting to Toronto seemed to me the beginning of my reaffirmation of this approach. To be in Toronto for 6 months meant the world to me at this point in Melanie's life, and I was determined to make the very most of the opportunity.

By the end of June, a pattern was emerging, and I was laying definite plans for activities that I would begin in September when the school year would reopen. First, the OCCC had made it clear that they intended to offer Melanie and myself every support available for the period of our temporary residence. Since Clive would be working, our OHIP (Ontario Hospital Insurance Plan) would become effective, which would stand the cost of weekly therapy sessions for Melanie as well as my own enrollment in a weekly counseling program for parents.

All this seemed too good to be true! An opportunity to participate in guided group discussion with parents going through the same experience as I, the availability of a small library on the subject of children with disabilities, the chance to be taught methods of helping my beautiful Little Bird, and the chance for her to be handled and taught by persons other than me who were trained and experienced in helping children like her.

As I leaped at the opportunities, I grieved for all the parents in Trinidad and other places who would never know the comfort and encouragement to be gained from such services—services provided by the state for citizens with disabilities and their families. I promised myself that I would work toward bringing about such services when I returned home.

In addition, I was laying plans for helping myself by practical experience. I had obtained permission to work as a volunteer in the OCCC school as of September and had already visited a number of classes in order to help me decide at what level I would like to work. Of course, I was most interested in Melanie's level and quickly gravitated toward a couple of classes known as the developmental classes. Here teachers and volunteers worked on stimulating awareness and response in about eight young children with very severe disabilities.

All the children had physical and apparently intellectual disabilities to the extent that, at the age of 4, very few of them could sit independently and none had speech. This was an entirely new world for me. Shaken as I was by the sight of these children with severe disabilities, I felt a driving need to come to grips with their situation and to develop the skills, emotional and otherwise, that would be necessary to help them.

The head teacher of these two small groups was a young woman named Martha. Her cheerful and positive manner set the tone for the group, and as I watched her admiringly, I could not know how central a role she would one day play in Melanie's and my life.

Meanwhile, Sick Kids' Hospital was also pursuing further investigations of Melanie's condition. Dr. Pape had suggested three follow-up referrals: an appointment with an eye doctor with the fancy title of neuro-ophthalmologist (this meant an eye specialist who had studied the links between the eyes and the central nervous system); appointments with the radiology department to study Melanie's swallowing mechanism as well as her skull and jaw by means of X-ray; and last but by no means least, an appointment with a therapist who would give me advice on feeding.

Of all of these, the most startling and the most revealing was the esophageal motility study. This turned out to be an X-ray of the actual process of swallowing taking place in Melanie's esophagus. It was accomplished by mixing some barium into Melanie's food and having her swallow it while an X-ray tracked the progress of the barium.

I fed Melanie in my usual fashion and sat in total amazement as the movement of the barium down my little girl's throat was projected onto a television screen. I was overwhelmed by what this miraculous product of man's imagination was able to tell us about the inadequacy of Melanie's feeding mechanism. As the colored liquid made its very shaky way down her little throat, the radiologist explained three things that were happening.

First, the liquid was progressing in irregular fits and starts because of poorly coordinated peristaltic waves within the esophagus. *Peristalsis,* I learned, is a term that refers to the normally rhythmic and powerful push of the muscles of the entire feeding system, which force food through the esophagus, stomach, and bowel. In Melanie's case, these muscles, like all the others in her body, just did not work right!

I sat quietly and, for once, speechless as the doctor continued. He pointed out that in addition to the weak peristalsis, her soft palate seemed also to be poorly coordinated, which resulted in the reflux of liquid into the nasal area. Further, and more worrying, was the fact that small quantities of the fluid were being aspirated, that is, going into her lungs; her frequent coughing was in response to this but was not always strong enough to clear the trachea.

So at last we had a clear and indisputable explanation of Melanie's constant coughing, choking, and vomiting. The picture explained also her continuing discomfort and fretfulness after feeding, as it was evident that some of the fluid remained in her esophagus for a prolonged period of time.

This first look into the inside of Melanie's body was very painful for me—painful yet so helpful in terms of improving my understanding of this unique little person. How far-reaching were the effects of this terrible thing that had happened to Melanie? How much more would there be to learn about this outwardly beautiful little body whose control center had gone so awry?

The other Sick Kids' referrals were less dramatic than this one but also helpful. The skull and jaw X-rays revealed no structural abnormalities, leaving us to assume that the tightness of Melanie's jaws was indeed a result of spasticity.

Dr. Berry, the eye specialist, could not discover anything more revealing than Dr. Pape's observations, but one new development did take place in the course of his examination. Melanie, for the first time that I had seen, actually did move her eyes in order to follow his moving of a bright-red striped cloth. With her head being held steady by me, and what must have been a great desire on her part to see more of the gaudy material, Melanie showed that she could force those eyes out of their habitually fixed position! This was a start and something to work on in the future.

Dr. Berry also observed the beginning of a squint, that is, that her eyes were not always centered, one tending to drift at an abnormal angle. He spoke of the possibility of surgery in the future to correct this condition.

The last two of Dr. Pape's referrals were the beginning of our relationship with two professionals who were to play a constructive and central part in Melanie's treatment. Dr. Saul Greenberg was to be her general pediatrician from that point on, since Dr. Pape felt it unfair to my brother Philip to continue to be responsible for the ongoing problems of a little niece so beloved yet so worrying. Soon, Dr. Greenberg's phone number would become the best-known number in our home.

Sarah Blacha was my last and, as it turned out, most long-lasting referral. The name seemed familiar, but it was not until I met her that I recalled that I had noticed the name written on the front cover of a booklet on the handling of children with cerebral palsy, which my friend Cathy had sent to me in Trinidad some months before. The same booklet had also been sent by Philip. (Cathy apparently had harassed the Sick Kids' therapists for reading material for me, while Philip had made himself a familiar pest at OCCC.)

So there we were, in Sarah Blacha's office, seeking advice on feeding for my Little Bird. Sarah's name would become a household word for us, as this was the beginning of a long and unequivocally supportive relationship not only for me but for Melanie as well.

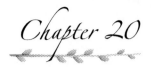

Chapter 20

INVISIBLE CHAINS

Summer was upon us, and as the city swung into the mood of abandon customary to that season, I settled into our new phase with an increasing sense of unreality.

Not having been through the previous winter and spring, and being accustomed by then to perpetual summertime, I had no outer shackles to throw off. The physical freedom that brings such release after months of overcoats and boots meant nothing to me, so I could not identify even on the most superficial level with the mood of the city.

The initial period of excitement and discovery of Melanie's problems was over, and by the beginning of July we had moved into a one-bedroom apartment conveniently located near St. Clair and Yonge. Near the subway, stores, cinemas, and a small park, the location was ideal for allowing Melanie and me some freedom of movement.

But our shackles were within. Deep in the center of my beautiful Little Bird were the invisible chains that constrained her to a life so circumscribed, so limited—chains that bound us together. By now, the symbolic lizard of my early dream was almost always out of sight, and I grew from strength to strength in loving Melanie.

It was the incredibly unique demands of this love that made me feel so separate from the world. I can remember a rare opportunity to go shopping without her one day, wandering through the new, ever-so-sophisticated subway shopping mall at Bloor and Yonge, at the heart of this city I had remembered so fondly, and feeling only a profound sense of alienation from it all— the fluorescent lights, the steel and plastic decor, the vast display of vivacious, skimpy summer wear. I could see nothing that appealed to me, no one in the swirling crowds who seemed real. Here was my dream of the staircase come true. All I could see in my mind's eye was Melanie—Melanie, so different from all this, so much more beautiful and yet so flawed, and a life in which the glamour flaunted here could have no meaning.

Of course, apart from any philosophical or emotional constraints, the practicalities of our days dictated my mood, and perhaps my sense of alienation was what enabled me to do what had to be done. For the summer was long and difficult. After such a wonderful start, the Nestargel, which had been so effective in keeping Melanie's food down, was becoming less successful. Her vomiting was increasing and her weight was at a standstill. Worse, she was developing a pattern of running a fever quite regularly and often appearing to be extraordinarily tense, with teeth clenched, her little body trembling. Dr. Greenberg wondered if she was having seizures, but one criterion did not fit: she could be distracted from this behavior when picked up and talked to, and we were told that in a seizure, this would not be possible. I had never seen one but felt sure that this was not the problem.

The fevers became so frequent that at one point Dr. Greenberg hospitalized her overnight for observation. The blood tests showed no infection, and her one night in this world-famous hospital was enough to drive me into a state of intense anxiety, for I was convinced that I was the only person capable of feeding Melanie.

By now, Sarah, our feeding therapist, and Dr. Greenberg were recommending withdrawal of the Nestargel. It was true that it was not working as well as before, and they felt that overall her diet was really inadequate. The Nestargel, they argued, was only a thickening agent with no nutritive value, and it would be better to try to get her onto a more balanced diet.

So with some reluctance, I withdrew the Nestargel and started to aim for a diet of fluids thickened only by food supplements and pureed solid foods. Sarah thought of everything. We must have tried every baby food on the shelf and, finally in great excitement, discovered that pureed meat would stay down absolutely. Melanie just never vomited the meat. It was the first and only substance that seemed heavy enough to defy those jumpy esophageal muscles. Dr. Greenberg was pleased but warned that she must retain enough fluid to flush the salts out of her system. I realized the importance of this but did not then understand the terrible implications of this warning. And so we struggled through the summer, the vomiting, it seemed, getting worse than ever except for the consistently successful meat puree and certain pureed fruits that seemed to stay down reasonably well. At the end of June, Melanie had been weighing 9 pounds and 12 ounces, and now, nearing the end of August, she was down to 9 pounds and 4 ounces. All I could think was that here she was close to her first birthday, weighing little more than the average newborn.

It had been a long and difficult summer, but in spite of this deteriorated feeding and weight loss, Melanie had made two significant strides—she had begun reaching out physically for the world and was showing improvement in her eye control.

The first toy Melanie ever reached out for was a spiky, squeaky blue porcupine offered to her in a therapy session at OCCC. As she stretched out her left hand for the toy, I felt a leap of joy and affirmation. She did care about the world and would be able to reach for it, however clumsily. Further, she was beginning to bring her hands together in front of her body and play with them. This apparently simple discovery of her own hands was more than just a sign of self-awareness that the average baby goes through at about 4 months of age. With Melanie, it also brought the relief of knowing that she was physically capable of bringing her hands to the midline of her body, which, the therapists explained, was a motor task that babies with cerebral palsy often have great difficulty doing.

Melanie's early attempts at eye-tracking were stimulated by Clive's 17-year-old son by his former marriage. Robert-Clive had come from New York to visit us and had fallen in love with his new little sister. His favorite activity with her was holding her head still while moving his face from left to right in front of her. To our delight, she would slowly force her eyes across, from side to side, once, twice, maybe three times, in pursuit of Robert's smiling face.

Melanie was still vomiting and grossly underweight, but by the end of the summer there was no doubt that she was responding more and more to her environment. Early in September, she began reaching for my face, and at last, it was clear that our relationship would be truly reciprocal. The rewards had begun to come and, with them, a greater motivation than ever to do everything possible for Melanie.

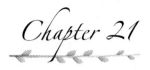

Chapter 21

LOVE AND FAITH

September came with its gradual change from green to the browns, yellows, and deep reds of autumn. A year had passed since Melanie had burst into our world, changing our lives so drastically. A year of anxiety and exhaustion dotted here and there with brief yet overwhelming moments of joy.

One such moment occurred on the night of September 16th, almost a year to the date that I had first looked at Melanie with doubt and fear, aware of the possibility that I could actually resent this vulnerable little creature, so delicate yet so powerful in her ability to change the course of my life.

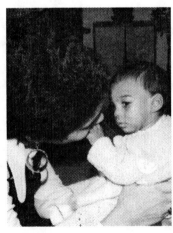

One year old, reaching for Mummy's face

I sat with her on my lap that night, a week before her birthday, and as she reached for my face, I was overwhelmed by a sense of intense communication with her—a current of mutual acknowledgment and love that passed between us. And I knew that my season of doubt was over.

I recorded my feelings that night and will transcribe them verbatim here:

Now, at this very late stage, I have decided to believe in Melanie. Oh, my beautiful Baby Bird, I do believe in you. Something in your eyes tonight said please, please, please, here I am! And after a year of loving you, I knew who you were. I know who you are.

Tonight for the first time that I can recall, I cried for you for the pain that you were experiencing from sluggish bowels. I cried for your pain rather than my own. I do believe this was a first for me.

Perhaps you will really be a person for me now. I saw that person reaching for my face tonight—a person, instead of a flawed piece of myself, which must either be fixed or cast out (if thine eye offend thee, pluck it out).

Even as I write this, the first time I have felt the need to record my feelings for you, I wonder if it is true and feel the old skepticism and doubt threaten. But I know I have made a start.

To you, my darling Melanie, my love and faith.

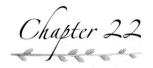

MUMMY THERAPY

Of one thing I was sure: this little girl knew me, and she knew her Daddy. Her usual manner of greeting me was with a cry and a start. Her smiles were still reserved for whistles (I had learned to whistle, too!) and a few other specific stimuli such as having her face blown on or being wheeled around rapidly.

By her 1st birthday, Melanie's motor control had also improved, and her birthday picture shows a rather sad looking little girl managing to sit fairly upright, supported firmly at the waist by Mummy's half-hidden hands.

I say sad looking because this was a feature that was beginning to worry me. She was not so much sad as quiet. Despite her increasing awareness, Melanie seemed to be having frequent periods of unusual quietness, no smiles, less rolling around, and most noticeably, no crying and very few sounds. This was very noticeable in a little girl who had always been very vocal, and neither the medical personnel nor I could imagine what was wrong.

But September brought many changes, and the busy schedule I set for myself helped me to contain my anxiety. I was due to begin regular volunteer work at OCCC as planned but still did not know who would keep Melanie while I rushed up to the center in between feedings. One day, Danny, one of the OCCC therapists, gave me quite the shock of my life by informing me that the center would be sending me a babysitter one day a week. Mrs. Marshall would come every Monday, she said, from 8:00 a.m. to 4:00 p.m., and would care for Melanie all day while I did whatever I pleased; I had never dreamed of such a service, of someone experienced in handling children with cerebral palsy coming to relieve me of what had become the all-consuming responsibility of my life. And it worked! Mrs. Marshall, a pleasant, gentle lady of middle age, arrived faithfully every Monday morning to do my job for me. I was determined to make the most of this and soon doubled up my plans for volunteer work. I would go on Monday mornings to the Centennial Nursery School program for preschoolers with disabilities in the basement of a nearby church and, in the afternoon, to Martha's class at OCCC. Soon, I was confident enough to look for another babysitter and found just the person, a graduate student in special education named Barb McKay, who came on Thursday afternoon while I went once more to OCCC.

Therapists and friends kept saying, "Why do three volunteer sessions a week, why not take some of that time for yourself?" But this *was* for me. My aim was to learn all I could about working with these children because I already knew that the day would come when I would be teaching children with disabilities besides Melanie.

So Mondays and Thursdays were volunteer work, and Wednesday mornings were set aside for Melanie's and my therapy. The PIS (Parents Information Services) program at OCCC included an hour with children, parents, and therapists together and an hour of discussion for parents while the children were babysat. Special arrangements were made for Melanie to have individual therapy in the first hour, however, in keeping with what seemed to me OCCC's policy of extra-special help for their visiting client from Trinidad.

In addition to all this, I made another decision that now seems to me quite astounding in terms of how much I was trying to do under very difficult circumstances. I allowed Georgia to talk me into applying to teach a night course for adults at Centennial

Community College. Since I had been a lecturer in English there from 1971 to 1973, it was relatively easy for me to get the job. Georgia convinced me that this would be by far the best therapy for me, and I agreed although somewhat fearfully.

Looking back, I can see how intensive my program was of personal therapy that fall. I attended physical therapy sessions with Melanie, group discussions with other parents, volunteer work, teaching a college course in English, while all the time I was dealing with Melanie's early rising, night waking, and interminable feeding and vomiting. It was therapy by stimulation and exhaustion. I was tired, but I loved the variety and interest these activities brought me as well as the increasing awareness of the world of disability, a world I had known nothing of a year before.

Indeed, by mid-Fall, my sense of alienation had gone. I had returned to the world with new eyes and new antennae and with a renewed confidence and sense of hope, despite the frustration of Melanie's continuing feeding difficulties.

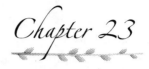

A VERY SICK BABY

It was fortunate that I had passed a crucial stage in my own personal response to Melanie, for unknown to me she was heading for a crisis that could have taken her life. The periods of quietness that I had started noticing in September were growing more frequent, and by early November, there were almost no sounds to be heard from my usually noisy Little Bird, and very few smiles. Neither the doctor nor I could think what was causing this quietness; indeed, what was becoming almost lethargy.

Somewhere in September, her vomiting had become so severe that Dr. Greenberg, Sarah, and I had finally decided that we would try tube feeding, the idea being that in bypassing the spastic esophageal muscles, the fluids might stay down better.

A year earlier, I had been horrified by the sight of the hated nasal feeding tube and could not be present when it was being inserted by the nurses. One year later, here I was, prepared to learn to insert the tube myself.

Sarah arranged two sessions with a nurse at Sick Kids' who would teach me the procedure. Although terrified at first, I quickly mastered the procedure of inserting the tube either orally or nasally, testing to be sure it was in her stomach and not in her lung, then pouring the fluid in. Since we did not want to leave the tube in, I used the oral procedure in which the tube was inserted through her mouth and removed immediately after the feeding. My fear of hurting Melanie subsided quickly as she made only small objections at first and soon began to cooperate quite well.

So for a month or so I had been using the tube feeding for most of her fluid feedings, with the other meals consisting mainly of pureed meat and fruits. The fluids sometimes stayed down a little better with the tube, but it was not at all consistent. I had taken to holding a 1-ounce cup to her mouth to collect what she brought up, and there were times when she regurgitated more than I had put in.

Yet I had not linked the poor fluid retention to Melanie's increasing quietness and lethargy. I had been advised to watch for certain signs of dehydration, such as looseness of the skin, dry mouth, and sunken eyes, but did not see these occurring except for increasingly dark circles under her eyes, which she had always had a tendency toward.

One day, in mid-November, Sarah came on a home visit to demonstrate to me how to stimulate chewing using pieces of chocolate or cheese. We were also trying to experiment with a variety of foods to see what might stay down better. But the session went very badly, Melanie showing almost no response to anything we did and simply falling asleep on the chocolate. Both Sarah and I were very worried at her extreme tiredness but still did not know what to make of it. That was Wednesday, and Clive had gone to New York on business for 3 days, planning to spend the weekend with his brother and return on Sunday.

On Thursday morning, November 12th, Melanie did not wake up at her usual 7 o'clock. I puttered around the apartment, glad for the opportunity to do a few things for myself before having to attend to her feeding.

At 8 o'clock, she was still sleeping, and I thought I would give her a few more minutes since we had a therapy session planned for that morning. In all her life, I had never had to wake Melanie in the mornings—she was *always* up before me and, in fact, had become my alarm clock. So at about 8:30 a.m., I decided she must not be well, and I had better wake her. I leaned over her crib, saying her name, but got no response. I gave her a gentle shake—no response. As I lifted one arm, the normally stiff little limb flopped back into placed like a blob of jelly.

Something was terribly wrong, and I picked her up, calling her name loudly. As I gathered the limp little body into my arms, her eyes flickered open for a moment, slid over to one side, then closed.

I thought, *she's in a coma! Sick Kids' Hospital!*

I threw her into her car seat and drove as I never had before. I could not know then that this would be but a foreshadowing of another drive I would have to make for Melanie years later. I rushed into the emergency department at 555 University Avenue, an address I can never forget. Within 15 minutes, there was an intravenous drip in her arm, blood samples were being taken, and preparations being made to take her, drip and all, to radiology for a chest X-ray.

The wait seemed interminable. I can remember sitting in a corridor somewhere in that vast hospital, struggling to keep myself under control and looking up to see Dr. Greenberg's usually calm face now tense and anxious coming toward me. Having just arrived, he knew only that Melanie had been hospitalized. He said, "What happened?"

I blurted, close to incoherence, "Oh, she's sick! She's very sick!"

And he responded, meaninglessly, "When did she get sick?"

I felt a surge of gratitude at the tone of absolute concern that marked every aspect of his response; I realized that he had caught my panic and was thrown momentarily off his usual professional balance. As I watched him go off to check on the test results, I knew that whatever ward they would put her in and however many specialists would examine her, Melanie would have a friend in this huge hospital.

By noon Dr. Greenberg was able to give me the diagnosis and tried to put into perspective the pattern of the last few months. Melanie was suffering from a severe electrolyte imbalance. This meant that the chemical balance of her body was seriously disturbed, owing to a massive buildup of sodium in her system. With insufficient fluid being retained, the kidneys simply could not do their work of flushing out the excess salts derived from the solid part of her diet. The way I understand it, the condition was related to, but not necessarily the same as, dehydration. Dr. Greenberg agreed that there were no serious superficial signs of dehydration such as I had been looking for, but dehydration was part of the condition.

This was the most serious problem revealed by the tests. The only treatment for it would be very gradual reintroduction of fluids into her system through intravenous feeding, and it could be days before they might be sure that she would recover unharmed. A secondary problem was pneumonia caused by aspiration—that is, she had inhaled some of the feeding into her lung, and this had created an infection. This would be treated by antibiotics, also given intravenously, and should clear up within 2 weeks.

I was assailed by a feeling of guilt and failure. How could I, with all my careful measuring of feedings, collecting of vomit, and insertion of tubes, have failed to realize that she simply was not keeping down enough fluid? How could Melanie have been getting sicker before my very eyes and I not realize what was happening?

Besides my talk with Dr. Greenberg, two other conversations of that day stand out in my memory, both also with doctors. The first conversation was with the senior resident in charge of the ward she was placed in. When the endless routines and red tape for admission had been completed and Melanie finally installed in a ward called the Sick Room with only four children and two nurses, the time had come for me to leave. It was around 8:00 p.m., and I felt as though I had been lying under a steamroller all day.

Reluctantly, I prepared to go, and the resident came to speak to me. Very gravely and gently, he said, "Mrs. Teelucksingh, I must explain to you that your baby is very sick."

I said, "I know."

But he reiterated, "No, I mean she is seriously ill. We cannot guarantee that she will get better."

With a sinking heart, I listened to his detailed explanation of the intravenous procedure that was being used, its potential for curing the condition, and its dangers.

I grieved for Melanie as I left the hospital that night. Georgia had persuaded me to go to dinner and when we got to the restaurant, I went directly to a pay phone to call my brother Philip. We had a long conversation in which I described all the medical details as well as my terrible sense of failure.

Philip's closing words gave me the perspective I needed. He said, "Bee, don't blame yourself. You've tried everything possible, and you've been wonderful. You've done everything in your power. It's time for someone else to try now. Accept what has happened, and give the responsibility over to the doctors. Let them try!"

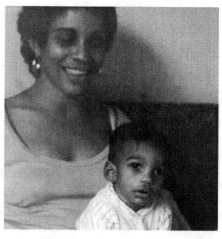

Fourteen months, a very sick baby

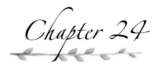

Chapter 24

THE TURNING POINT

Clive flew back from New York the next day, cutting his stay short, and together we began a month of watching and waiting. Of that month, the first week was the most harrowing for me, as I found myself in the unaccustomed role of helpless spectator as Melanie gradually returned to life. Within 48 hours the intravenous rehydration process had achieved the brunt of its miraculous work, bringing the chemical balance of Melanie's body back within normal limits although the process would not be perfect for a week or so.

Melanie's awareness was returning gradually, and on about the 4th morning, as I walked into the ward entering through a door directly in her line of vision, my Little Bird responded immediately with her jerky start, eyes filling with tears, and the little mouth puckered to make the only sound she knew how—
ooooo.

Melanie was back with us and, like any other child in hospital, was simultaneously glad to see her Mummy and yet angry at having been betrayed into the hands of strangers in sterile white coats. Within another day or so, she was also beginning to show her annoyance at the physical constraints of the intravenous tubing, her hands strapped down to the bed to ensure the security of the needle in the tiny veins. From time to time, her struggles would result in the needle slipping out, only to be replaced in another spot, varying from waist to ankle and on occasion even to her temple.

So Melanie was engulfed in tubes, the intravenous ones continuing the process of rehydration and also feeding antibiotic medication directly into her bloodstream to combat the aspiration pneumonia. Meanwhile the naso-gastric tubes were permanently in place for all her feeding. Within a week, the life-endangering electrolyte imbalance had been fully corrected, but it would be another week before the pneumonia would be cleared up.

But Dr. Greenberg was concerned about the root cause of this terrible crisis in Melanie's life. What could be done to improve her feeding system to ensure that this would not happen again? His decision was to keep her in the hospital to enable a thorough study of the problem through observation and the trial of various foods and medications. I cannot describe how grateful I was for this approach. Philip had been right—it was their turn to try, and this experienced medical team would do all in its power to solve the problem of Melanie's continuing failure to thrive.

It was a challenging month of tubes, formulas, and medications. The challenge for the dietician was to come up with a liquid formula composed of all the nutrients needed in an appropriate balance, watery enough to provide adequate fluid and to go through the tube but thick enough to be likely to stay down. This was no easy task, and in fact, it simply did not succeed. Even the thickest possible consistency proved too light to resist Melanie's jumpy peristalsis, and the vomiting continued, more at some times than at others, inconsistent enough to allow a fluctuating pattern of weight gain and loss over the weeks.

Along with the efforts of the dietician went the efforts of the gastroenterologist and various other "ologists" too numerous to mention, and indeed, to remember! A number of medications were tried, all aiming at altering the muscle tone of the stomach and esophagus in order to allow a more steady flow of food.

One of the biggest problems, of course, was to ensure that the medication stayed down. There is not much point giving antivomit medication if the medication comes up with the vomit, and this was exactly what happened much of the time. The medical team contrived various methods to try to ascertain how much Melanie actually vomited and whether the medication had also come up. These included using a special absorbent bib that had been preweighed and would be weighed after the vomiting subsided, and at one point, an inventive head nurse decided to color the medication artificially so that any sign of bright blue on the bib would be recognized as medication.

They certainly did try! After 2 or 3 weeks, some of the specialists even discussed with me a couple of extreme medical procedures that could, theoretically, be used in an extreme case of failure to thrive. These included a surgical procedure known as gastrostomy, which involved inserting a feeding tube directly into the child's stomach. This was quite unacceptable to me and to the specialist, as it seemed to render the child virtually an invalid.[1]

Another procedure discussed seemed to me, though to no one else, a real possibility as a last resort—the idea of intramuscular injection of a medication to ensure its absorption into the system. I felt that, as horrible as this would be for Melanie, if it was the only way to ensure her life and health, I would do it. But even the doctor who first mentioned it would not support the idea.

The fact that toward the end of the month this sort of solution was being discussed indicates how severe the problem was. Nothing they tried had really worked, it seemed, although by this time, Melanie was showing an overall weight gain of perhaps 6 ounces despite a fluctuating daily and weekly pattern. It was still

---

[1] Twenty-five years later, this procedure is common practice and our refusal to use it seems incomprehensible to special educators who work with similarly affected children.

hard to tell whether any given medication had stayed down consistently, and when it had there was little reason to believe that it had decreased the vomiting.

By Melanie's 4th week in the hospital, the doctors were baffled and, it seemed, helpless. They had done all they could, and though she had gained a little weight, Melanie's pattern had not changed at all. There was really no more they could do. Melanie was now in good health, her life had been saved by the efficiency and up-to-date procedures of this world-renowned hospital, and once more, it was time for Clive and me to resume our responsibility for the continuing life and health of this delicate little creature we loved so much.

I was close to desperation. The worst thing I could imagine was having Melanie continue to be semi-invalid, at risk of dehydration or starvation for the rest of her life, and the constant state of anxiety in myself created by such a responsibility. She had learned so much in the past few months, was so much more aware of her environment, and so much more responsive and expressive, but if she could not eat, it would all be worth nothing.

I was puzzled by one fact, however. In the previous few months at home, she had gained no more than a few ounces, yet in her 4 weeks in the hospital, she had gained 6 ounces despite what seemed to be the same pattern of vomiting. Why?

The day before she was to leave, I sat chatting with a couple of Melanie's nurses. I made this observation to them, and as we talked, one of the nurses suddenly thought of something. She said, "You know, I notice that when I give her a feeding on my night shift and she's sleeping, it usually stays down."

My heart skipped. She was saying that feedings administered through the tube during Melanie's sleep usually stayed down. The other nurse agreed. I asked them over and over, "Are you sure?" If they were right, then the solution was before my eyes: I would simply feed her while she slept.

I would feed Melanie while she slept. I cannot overstate the importance of these words, of this discovery, for it would lead to the turning point in Melanie's life.

We left the hospital the next day about a week before Christmas, and I was overwhelmed with gratitude to the two nurses who had given me something to hold onto.

And it is on this point only that I can fault the procedures of this efficient, ultramodern hospital. Somewhere, in its maze of carefully planned schedules and shifts, there should have been room for every nurse involved in a case like this to see herself as an integral part of the problem-solving process, as a member of a team looking for answers rather than simply following instructions on schedule.

What I mean is that if any of the nurses attending Melanie had been asking their own questions regarding a solution to their patient's vomiting, they would surely have made this observation much earlier and to the persons in charge of her feeding program. As it was, it was simply a matter of chance that I fell into such a productive conversation the day before Melanie's discharge. But for this conversation, I would have gone home feeling as helpless as when I brought her in.

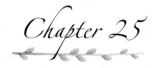

SLEEP FEEDING

I t was Christmas, the season of hope, and we were alive with hope. The new feeding approach was off with a bang. I was determined, Clive as always supportive, and Melanie cooperative.

Sarah, Melanie's feeding therapist, solved the problem of what to do with the tube while she slept. I simply pinned a mitten onto her shoulder and tucked the long tube in. The short tubes didn't work because she rolled a lot in her sleep, and adhesive tape alone did not keep it in place. Dr. Greenberg solved the problem of how to ensure that she slept through her night of feeding: an old fashioned sedative, chloral hydrate, with no barbiturate content or addictive qualities, did the job. And the dietitian solved the problem of what to feed her: Three fluid feedings at night, one of plain sugar water, and two of her special formula, ensured an adequate balance. In the day, Melanie had only small meals of crushed potato or meat, whatever would stay down, and frequent but tiny sips of water no more than a spoonful at a time. And it worked!

What timing! Clive's 6-month appointment in Toronto had run close to 9 months, and we were due to return to Trinidad the 1st or 2nd week in January.

By the appointed time for our departure, I had established a regular routine for Melanie's bedtime. After her story and hugs,

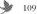

it was time to insert the nasal tube. As soon as the tube was in place, in went the chloral hydrate, and within minutes she was fast asleep.

The slow and steady breathing of sleep was the sign for Melanie's first balanced meal and first real drink for the day. Then just before my bedtime she received a long drink of water, and whenever my internal automatic clock woke me during the night, usually around 2:00 a.m., she had her second substantial though liquid meal. As soon as she woke in the morning, I removed the tube, and she could spend the day looking like any other pretty little girl, taking occasional small meals of semisolids and the occasional drink of one teaspoon of water or juice.

And so my hands were full but my heart light that Christmas.

What had we gained from our stay in Toronto? Almost at the last minute, and just in time, I had gained information on what had been the most crucial hurdle of Melanie's life. I anticipated returning to Trinidad with increased understanding and a new, if unconventional, feeding approach that I hoped would make the difference between living and existing for Melanie.

In addition, I had learned a great deal personally. In the counseling group at OCCC, I had gained a great deal of information and, through discussion with other parents, had discovered not only that we all shared the same fears and concerns, but above all that I could consider myself fortunate in the sort of family and social supports I had, as well as my own personal resources. In my volunteer work and therapy sessions, I had learned a lot about how to stimulate young children with disabilities and had been gratified by the support and encouragement I had received regarding my own handling of Melanie. Sarah, for example, had been so pleased with my interaction with Melanie that she invited us to be included in an educational film being made by the Canadian Institute on Mental Retardation. Our small role in the film was intended to model positive mother–child interaction.

Another thing that had boosted my confidence during our 9-month stay in my old home was simply the experience of seeing a wide variety of children with disabilities being treated with such respect and receiving the best in medical and therapeutic attention regardless of the severity of their disability. Indeed, some of the children in

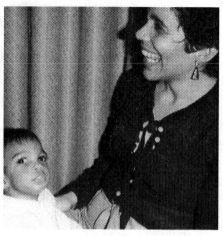

One year, four months: getting better!

the developmental class at OCCC represented the most extreme end of the spectrum of disabling conditions.

I remember in particular one little girl of 3 or 4 years, absolutely rigid in body, with no spontaneous movement, no vision, no hearing, and indeed, no show of response whatever except for a shiver when handled a lot and a most distressing, continuous rattle accompanying every breath she took. She was of a Portuguese family and, in the manner of that culture, was decked out as a proper little girl—beautiful dresses, long, impeccably braided hair, and sparkling gold rings, bracelets, and earrings. I wept when I learned that her name was Felisamena, meaning happiness.

I had much to be grateful for. My beautiful Little Bird could move, cry, smile, see, hear, recognize people, and above all, could show that she returned our love. And soon, I felt sure, she would be able to eat and grow healthy and strong.

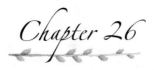

THRIVING

We returned to Trinidad via a short visit to my parents in Jamaica. It was there that Melanie's new feeding program suffered its first and only setback. For some reason, she started waking at night and bringing up the feeds, and within a couple of days, the symptoms of the electrolyte imbalance were setting in again—the quietness and lethargy that I had grown so accustomed to just a few months before.

We appealed to a pediatrician in charge of the Children's Hospital in Kingston, and this wonderful lady, as soon as she heard the history and saw Melanie, admitted her to the ward for a day and simply rehydrated her by intravenous feeding for the day.

That night Melanie slept through the night, and from then on, she never looked back! We arrived in Trinidad in mid-January, and within a week I knew for sure she was on the way up. The nighttime tube feedings were working like a charm. Somehow Melanie's feeding system simply worked best while she slept. I can only assume that the muscles of her esophagus and stomach were then relaxed enough to do their work smoothly.

It was 1977, and we were home! Melanie was thriving now, and I was beginning to feel once more intact as a person. With Melanie's health finally under control, I could turn some attention to what seemed to me the necessary next step in the therapeutic process for Clive and me, for our family as a whole—a second baby.

I felt that I could never fully recover my self-confidence as a woman and a mother unless I could have the experience of successful and healthy childbearing. I felt this essential for the reestablishment of my own self-image and for the healthy development of our family.

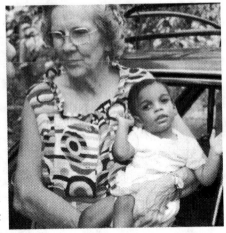

One year, four months, with Grandma in Jamaica

The kind of total attention absorbed by Melanie in our family had been inescapable up to now, but we knew that to continue that way would inevitably produce an emotionally lopsided family. We needed a change. We needed balance, the joy of an easier, more normal experience of parenting for Clive and me, and we needed a sibling for Melanie.

We had received genetic counseling in Toronto in which we had been assured that there was no reason to believe that there were any genetic factors at work in Melanie's condition. The history, and her condition, seemed to be certainly related to damage caused at the time of my hemorrhage at 10 weeks of gestation and the subsequent slow growth of the fetus. We were told that we should have no reason to expect problems with another baby.

Despite all this information and my overwhelming desire for another baby, I embarked on the new pregnancy in fear and trembling! Rationally, I did not expect problems, but on an imaginative level, my every fantasy was disastrous.

I found that I was unable to indulge in joyful and successful fantasies of the new baby. Every daydream of the coming event turned into a nightmare, and I simply could not envision the lovely, healthy baby I wanted so much.

But it was a wonderful, healthy pregnancy, and fortunately I was so busy with Melanie that I did not have much time to torture myself with horrible imaginings.

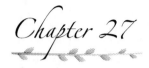

Chapter 27

NAMING THE WORLD

Sometimes from her eyes I have received fair speechless messages.

These words from Shakespeare's *The Merchant of Venice* capture exactly my sense of Melanie's communication with me. She spoke to me at all times with her eyes. In a face so perfectly formed, there was little muscular movement, hardly a raised eyebrow, frown, or grimace; in short, what amounted to very little variety of facial expression. Except for a beautiful, usually one-sided smile in response to certain favored stimuli, Melanie's face appeared beautiful but largely unresponsive.

Except for her eyes. To me, her eyes spoke the entire range of human awareness and response. There was interest, attentiveness, curiosity, joy, pain, annoyance, understanding, and love in those eyes, so bright and black like Jamaica's famous ackee seeds. *Ackee eyes,* we called them.

Melanie watched everything and everyone, moving her head to compensate for her poor eye control. To see her watch other children at play was a revelation. Turning her head with every toss of the ball, Melanie's head and eyes would appear to be at cross-purposes, the eyes finally arriving in correct focus only to find that the ball had already bounded off in another direction. Her head would immediately initiate its next attempt at participation in this game of incredible skill and coordination taken so for granted by its players.

114

As with my own incomprehension when Dr. Pape first explained Melanie's eye movements to me, her intention was not always evident to others. The best example I can give of this was the response of a little boy, Omar, at a birthday party where all the children were playing outside. I had put Melanie to stand in her walker near to the children, explaining that although she couldn't play she would enjoy watching them. After warning them not to bump into her, I took a seat with a group of other mothers on the patio, making sure that I could see the children's play.

After a few minutes, Omar came running in and assailed me in great frustration: "What's wrong with her?" he demanded. "Is she blind or what? She's not following the game!" As Omar's mother gasped in apology at her son's directness, I reacted with delight at the opportunity to explain my little girl to a child who cared enough to ask. Going outside with Omar, I explained to the children about Melanie's difficulty in redirecting her eyes, and demonstrated to them how she would turn her head in order to get her eyes into the right position to follow their play. Omar and his friends received this news with great excitement, and after testing my explanation by running back and forth in front of Melanie they devised a strategy to start calling out to her to try to give her advance warning of the direction in which they were going to throw the ball! As they shouted, "Melanie! Melanie! Look!" I returned to the adult group with great relief and we talked about how wonderful a child's honesty could be, how much more helpful than the pretenses of adults who hide their observations for fear of hurting another's feelings. Omar's openness gave me the opportunity to explain Melanie to her friends, opening the door for them to express their understanding and generosity.

So Melanie communicated with the world largely through her eyes. She was also very vocal, and I felt sure that if she could only have placed tongue and lips in the correct positions, what seemed to be noises would indeed have been words. She did have some limited variety of tone, so that one could tell if she was annoyed, pleased, or questioning, but because these were all throat noises with no lip, tongue, or jaw movement, her sounds seemed all the same and in general quite monotonous. But she certainly was noisy and made her presence felt by her combination of consistent though incomprehensible noises and those sparkling, compelling ackee eyes.

With these observations about her interest in her environment, and with her health and weight gain established, I knew it was time to pay serious attention to the development of her comprehension and, hopefully, communication.

I got the direction I needed from Nancy Finnie's book, *Handling the Young Cerebral Palsied Child at Home* (1975). In the chapter entitled *Speech,* I was struck by the following recommendation:

> Use the parts of his body, simple elementary toys, the things you use when feeding, bathing, dressing him and so on . . . . Use objects of different colors, shapes, textures and sounds even tastes and temperatures; name each of them and talk a little about them and what they are used for; all this will help to develop the sensory avenues that are necessary for the formulation of language. (Finnie, 1975, pp. 138–139)

This seemed such an obvious approach that I was amazed that I had not been doing it spontaneously. Of course, I was in the habit of talking to Melanie and usually kept up a sort of running commentary while handling her. From early infancy, her responsiveness to my voice had encouraged me to be at my talkative best with her. But my talk was simply affectionate chatter with no intention or attempt to teach. When I read Nancy Finnie's suggestions, I could not understand why I had not started talking to her in this more instructive and functional manner. Why had I not been doing the obvious elementary mothering activity of naming and explaining the world to my child?

The answer, it appears, is as simple as the question: I had assumed she was not ready for it. The reason for this became clear to me in reading an article by Mahoney and Seely (1976) titled "The Role of the Social Agent in Language Acquisition." The interaction of mother and child in language development was described as follows: "The modification of maternal speech depends partially upon the language of children, since maternal speech is more complex before children utter their first words than it is when they first utter two-word utterances" (Maloney & Sealey, p. 71).

Simply put, this means that in the normal process, a mother and infant mutually reinforce each other in communication. Thus, while the mother will at first use quite ordinary language with her infant, when the infant shows that she is ready to start talking the mother spontaneously begins to simplify her own speech so as to help the child's language development. Soon the mother is a spontaneous teacher of language and finds herself pointing, naming, repeating, correcting. In this way she simplifies the language-learning process for her child.

The mother of a child whose development is delayed is no different in principle. As long as her child performs like a baby, she interacts with her as a baby. Like other mothers, she responds to the baby's cues. The problem she faces is that her child may be very late in changing cues either because he or she is not ready or because he or she cannot demonstrate that readiness. In this situation, the mother of a child with a disability must work in the dark. She must work with minimal or no cues from her child. She must start at her child's fingertips, eyes, ears, nose, and tongue and work inward no matter how sparse the feedback. If the child is not ready, he will not learn, and his mother will experience considerable frustration. If he is ready, however, the rewards that await her are indescribable.

With this dawning realization, I started naming the world for Melanie, who, at 1 year and 6 months, had the size and behavior of an infant of about 4 months. At first, it felt a bit strange talking to her in measured words and tones intended for instruction, but since I was alone with her most of the day, my self-consciousness wore off quickly.

I decided to set specific objectives for her learning and set out first to teach her a response that I thought was probably the earliest gestural language babies display; that is, raising the arms to be picked up.

I started by saying, "Come to Mummy," with my arms outstretched, then putting *her* arms up, then picking her up immediately, saying, "Good girl, Melanie!" When I thought she seemed to be enjoying the routine, I started saying, "Come to Mummy," with my arms outstretched and simply waiting for her to respond. Upon the slightest appropriate response, even a movement of her arm, I would pick her up and praise her.

When I was sure that she was moving her arms in response to my words and gesture, I omitted the gesture and offered only the words, "Come to Mummy."

I started this routine in mid-March, and my notes give March 28th as the date I felt sure that Melanie had raised her arms in response to the verbal invitation alone. That is, I said, "Come to Mummy," *just* those words—no gesture—and she put her arms up to come.

It had taken her only 2 weeks to learn this, and I was overwhelmed. Obviously, she had been ready for this.

The next objective I set was for her to open her mouth in response to verbal encouragement while feeding. Up to then, I had become

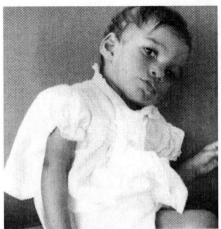

One year, five months, back home in Trinidad

accustomed to edging the spoon in and gradually forcing her to open her mouth enough to accommodate it.

Now I began holding the spoon in front of her mouth saying, "open" and not putting it in until she spontaneously opened. My notes give April 15th as the date on which I felt she was responding appropriately. She had certainly been ready also for this.

This fantastic start gave me the impetus I needed, and it was lucky that I had chosen these responses to start with, since after this the process went more slowly until about June when it picked up again.

During this time, I gained ideas from several sources. Some of the literature I found on teaching infants with disabilities suggested that special periods in the day be set aside for teaching, while others recommended an integration of all teaching into the daily routine with an emphasis on play. I used both approaches and soon began to feel like a teaching machine. I named and talked and pointed until it became second nature while Melanie sat in attendance on my every household activity.

The latter was accomplished by my pulling her around the house in her small umbrella pushchair. The kitchen was one of her favorite places, where she would sit in total attention to my stimulation of all her senses with bits of onion, sweet pepper, raw or cooked meat, fruits, and even handfuls of black pepper. The latter was her favorite, since she loved to sneeze and would follow each one with a huge smile and her squeal of delight.

From March to August of that wonderful year, Melanie grew from strength to strength in her comprehension of language, and my joy in her was matched only by the joy of knowing that the new life within me was growing stronger and healthier with every day, despite the inescapable fears of my imagination.

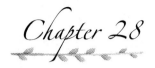

Chapter 28

MORNING HAS BROKEN

I think that the simplest way to give a picture of our successes and failures in those months is to transcribe from my diary the four pages on which I recorded some 5 months of work (see Figure 1). After our two early successes, there are no entries for the month of May, then several for June, July, and August.

Of all these entries, there is one on which I must comment because it represented for me a turning point in my perception of Melanie—the point at which I knew for sure that she would be able to make use of language at least receptively if not through speech.

Up until the end of June, all the responses Melanie was learning were responses to instructions, such as "Come," "Look at Mummy," and so on. Although I had been naming objects to her since March, I had not yet really tested her comprehension of the language involved. Toward the end of June, I noticed that whenever I put Melanie on her changing table, she would reach up to where her hair brush was kept just over her head and appear to make a swipe at the brush.

One day, as soon as I lay her on the table, I said, "Where is the brush, Melanie?" She reached up toward the brush. I sat her up in front of it and repeated the question again, and she reached for the brush, actually hitting it off the shelf. Disbelieving, I turned her around so that the brush was to her left and out of her line of vision;

Diary Entries

Participates in and enjoys social games (peek-a-boo, clap hands, etc.).	Smiles and squeals to "peek-a-boo" and other games, e.g., "up and down," "fall down."	July 1
	Smiles in response to names of songs.	July 20
	Opens hands for clapping.	August
Responds to instructions.	"Come to Mummy,"—arms outstretched.	March 28
	"Come here,"—rolls across room to Mummy.	June 15
	"Open your mouth,"—opens	April
	"Look at Mummy,"—turns, looks.	June
	"Touch," e.g., a toy.	July-August
	"Pull." "Push."	July-August
	"Open your fingers."	July-August
Responds to ritual phrases ("Pretty!" "Bye-bye").	Beginning to lift hand and wiggle fingers in response to "Bye-bye."	August 12
	Waves "Bye-bye."	End of August
Associates "Daddy," "Mummy" appropriately.	Turns, looks at Daddy in response to word.	June
	Turns, looks at Mummy in response to word.	July
Associates sounds with relevant objects (toys, door opening, car starting).	Reaches for correct object on hearing sound, e.g., squeaky toy, bell, music box.	Mid-June
	Turns appropriately on hearing door, car, footsteps.	July
Associates names with relevant objects (teddy, bell, ear, bed, water, etc.).	In response to the question "Where is the...?" turns, looks, and reaches for: brush, bed, eyes, nose, mouth, hair, water, soap	End of June
Associates names...	Ears, tongue, teeth, necklace, fingers, fridge, tree, book	End of July
	Milk, juice, spoon, dolly, bottle, comb, light, mirror, box, breast, car.	Mid-August
Gestures for communication.	Waves "Bye-bye."	End of August
	Raises hands on hearing "Come."	March
	Reaches for bottle at feeding time	June
Puts out hand for putting on blouse.	Pushes arm through sleeve.	August
Smiling.	Smiles at daddy's arrival home.	Mid-August
Face more relaxed and expressive.	Improving, more smiles—but...	July-August
Imitates syllable sounds.		
Makes syllable sounds in relation to people, objects.		

Figure 1.   Diary entries tracking Melanie's progress.

as soon as I asked the question again, she turned to the left and swung her right arm around directly to the brush. My heart leapt as I tested her, over and over, and she, appearing to enjoy the exercise, responded correctly every time.

I say that this was my turning point with Melanie because it meant to me that she was capable of taking part in the essentially human activity of identifying an object with a verbal symbol; she could understand language. I felt sure that if she could do that, she would be able to make sense of the world and live a meaningful life. I had never felt sure of that before.

During this time, one of my greatest joys was showing off Melanie's comprehension to all our friends, and she turned out to be as great a showoff as her mother. The very best of these occurrences was, to my intense gratification, the day she performed her "touching

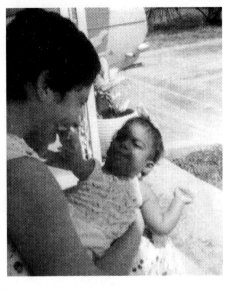

One year and nine months—learning to identify "eyes," "nose," and "mouth"

mouth, eyes, nose, ears" routine for our pediatrician, whose expectations of her had been so low a year earlier. Dr. McDowall, normally serious if not somber in manner, threw his head back and laughed in delight as I put my Little Bird through her paces. He made no attempt to conceal his surprise at her comprehension and congratulated me warmly on her progress.

During those months, Melanie made the final leap over the most crucial hurdle of her life—feeding. The tube-feeding regimen had worked consistently, and by June she was able to keep down enough fluid given by spoon during the day for me to eliminate one of the night feedings. My aim was to eliminate the tube feeding entirely by September in the hope that I would not have two babies to wake up to at night when October came.

But the improvement in Melanie's feeding system exceeded my expectations by 2 months. By June, the pattern was evident— the more fluid she kept down at nights through the tube feeding, the more weight she gained. The more weight she gained, the more fluid she was able to keep down by normal feeding during the day. In other words, the heavier she got, the less she vomited, and the less tube feeding was necessary.

One day in July, my friend Shirley, who for some months had been a great support and encouragement in my handling of Melanie, said, "Beth, you can stop the tube feeding now, she can take it all by mouth in the day." I responded that I might stop in a couple of weeks' time. Shirley, forever dictatorial, repeated, "Stop now—tonight." She took my feeding tubes, got into her car, and drove off!

And that was it. It was over—the nightmare of tubes and formulas, of adhesive tape and chloral hydrate, and the tension I felt every time I inserted the hated yet miraculous tube. Morning had broken. Melanie was alive and beautiful and thriving. She was aware and alert and involved in her world. She loved and was loved in return, and Clive and I awaited eagerly the new life that would make our family a full and normally functioning unit.

It was the summer of 1977, and we were on our way.

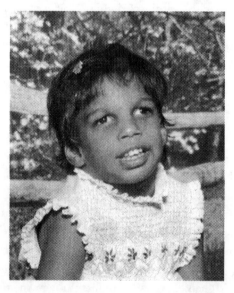

Age 2, growing up!

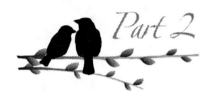

Part 2

Chapter 29

MARK

On October 18 of that year, at 4 o'clock in the morning, I made my first entry in a little diary that I call *The Book of Joy*. The entry reads:

The book of joy begins with tears
wild, trembling, overpowering
tears of joy that wash away the fear, the pain
now it is safe to cry
now cry
now weep the flood of fear
that filled the bed
that soaked the banks
now let it flow, now wash
now cleanse, now heal
now free

Mark had arrived—the world's oldest miracle reenacted for me, and as he left me, forcing his way into the world, I heard a voice like mine calling out as from a distance, "Is he all right? Is he all right? Is he all right?" Then uncontrollable tears, then laughter, then both becoming one as my son, screaming his newborn power, gave me his answer.

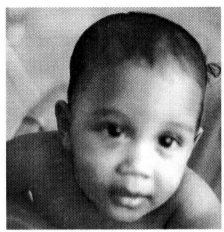

Mark at 3 months

As the days passed, and I gradually returned from my trembling euphoria, Mark introduced himself to me in no uncertain terms. I could hardly believe this was supposed to be the same experience I had known 2 years before in bearing my first child. This child's power overwhelmed me, and to me, he seemed no helpless human infant but rather a magnificent bundle of infinitely powerful instincts and reflexes, capable of commanding and making use of every ounce of available attention and sustenance.

In Melanie, I had seen true helplessness, a frail, beautiful little creature—a bird with a broken wing. And now I was awed by the power of this new creature we had made, an organism perfectly equipped for coping with life and motivated only by his own need for survival. I called him the Critter! To me, he seemed such an ornery little critter that in the first weeks I often feared that I would be unable to love him. How could one genuinely love a creature to whom one had to be so totally subservient! There was no doubt that he was the master, and I had neither the philosophy nor the energy to enter into a battle of wills with him.

For 3 months he was a colicky, screaming infant with a voice of thunder, and my condition moved rapidly from euphoria to exhaustion. There were days when every scream seemed an accusation against which I might have to defend myself, and of course one invariably resents one's accuser! Ah! My little Critter! In those early weeks how I loved and feared you! Melanie,

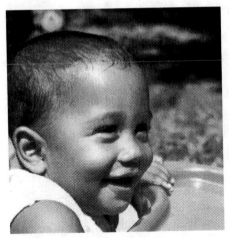

Mark at 3 months

meanwhile, was extremely impatient and resentful of this terrifying intruder into her peaceful Mummy-filled world. She drank an awful lot of milk in those months, since it was the only way I could quiet her extremely noisy resentment of the nursing procedure. Had I not been so exhausted, I might have been able to laugh at the sight of an overweight, distraught mother sitting on a couch holding a gobbling infant to her left breast while thrusting a bottle into the mouth of a small child sitting to the right in a green pushchair.

Clive kept saying that Mark would become calmer when he could move around independently, and his prophecy proved correct. Dr. McDowall, meanwhile, had predicted on the basis of Mark's alertness and perfect reflexes at birth that he would be bright and advanced in his development, and, sure enough, by 4 months he was moving around the entire room by rolling and wriggling, and at 5 months, he was up on all fours in a perfect 7-month-old crawl. As he gained in independence and mobility and could express his characteristic driving energy through movement and interaction with his environment, he became no longer the Critter but a true creature of delight.

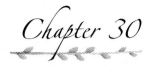

Chapter 30

SEEKING ANOTHER VIEW

When Mark was about 6 months old, Clive was offered the opportunity of participating in a work-related course in Barbados for 2 months.

I was delighted for him but knew I could not possibly survive in a house alone with the children for that length of time, so I solved the problem by deciding to go to my parents in Jamaica. This was an appealing opportunity for me, although not as simple as it sounds, since my father was by then bedridden and deteriorating steadily and my mother's hands were full to overflowing. I decided that I would go anyway, and Mummy and I would simply overflow together.

Above all, I was glad for an opportunity to be with my father, who in all my growing years had been my hero and the love of my life. It was painful to see that he could not interact with and perhaps not even recognize his grandchildren, but it was fulfilling just to be with him and to observe and participate in my mother's impeccable caring for him.

This visit, however, led to a crucial and painful event centering on Melanie. Everyone was tremendously impressed with Melanie's development in the year and a half since they had seen her. Mummy was so impressed that she suggested that it might be time for a reevaluation of her development and offered to pay our way to Toronto for this purpose. I had done so much work with her in that year and a half and had seen her transform from a limp creature with sunken eyes and regurgitated food streaming from both mouth and nose into a healthy little girl who, despite her slow facial responses and awkward movements, showed distinct interest in and awareness of her environment. I felt sure that anyone assessing her would also see the magnificent transformation, as did all our friends and family.

I was convinced by then that Melanie at $2^3/_4$ years had good intelligence, understood as much of what was going on as the average 2-year-old, and was hampered mainly by a tremendous motor disability that rendered jaw, facial, and eye movements as well as arms, and to a lesser extent, leg movements very difficult for her to accomplish. She could roll and would roll the entire length of the house to find someone if she had been left alone in the living room, for example. She would reach readily for objects of interest but would most often miss, appearing to misjudge the distance of the object. She had next to no grasp whatever, never holding an object for more than a few seconds, and if she was trying at the same time to move the arm, she would immediately release her hand grasp.

Overall, she seemed incapable of doing two things at a time. She could hold an object but not also move her arm. She could move her head or eyes but not both together. She could sit independently for a few moments but would lose her balance and topple the moment she tried to turn her head. She could suck on food and swallow it, but if she tried to vocalize during this process, the rhythm of her breathing and swallowing would go awry and she would choke on the food. The latter, of course, made her feedings still precarious, and I had developed a kind of symbiotic interaction at these times in which I would breathe with her, losing the rhythm simultaneously with her and thus actually anticipating the choke before it occurred.

In sum, I saw Melanie's muscular problem as essentially one of poor coordination of all her muscles and what should have been automatic systems. I was sure that the comprehension was there, its expression prevented only by the brain's inability to tell the muscles what to do. The diagnosis, as far as I was concerned, was some kind of pretty severe cerebral palsy. It was with this kind of outlook that I made arrangements for an assessment appointment at OCCC that June. Toronto was easy for me because of my network of supports there. I did try for an appointment with Dr. Challenor at Blythedale, who had been so encouraging, but she was not available at the time I planned, and I settled on OCCC.

So after 5 weeks with my parents in Jamaica, our little trio set out for Toronto in hopeful search of confirmation of my impression of Melanie's progress.

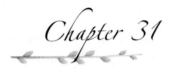

Chapter 31

THE FOREST OR THE TREES?

"**G**ross global brain damage with severe mental retardation." What more was there to say? "Gross global brain damage with severe mental retardation." The summary words of Dr. Wilmington's diagnosis rang through my ears like a death knell for Melanie. I was devastated and disbelieving. They could not be right, for her intelligence communicated itself to me at every turn. They could not be right because she had learned too quickly all the things I had tried to teach her. They could not be right because her eyes told me they were wrong. They could not, please God, be right because if they were, she would live a life so limited as to be almost useless. They could not be right because she was *my child!*

How does a mother tread the fine line between what she sees and what she wants to see in her child? Where are the strengths and where are the weaknesses of the objective view of the outsider, as compared with the subjective view of the mother?

I believe that the mother's advantage is that of intimacy, which allows her a depth of perception unavailable to an outsider. I knew, for example, that Melanie's difficulty in focusing her eyes often made her appear to be turning away from people when she was in fact trying to look at them. With the advantage of intimacy, I knew also that the little squeal that others might interpret as a cry was Melanie's version of a laugh. I knew that flared nostrils followed by a little yawn meant that she was emptying her bladder.

But the mother's intimacy may also be a disadvantage. That intimacy made it impossible for me to see Melanie for the first time—to see her in her totality as a functioning individual who exists in the present and who compares in any given way to other individuals.

Such intimate knowledge of my child, and in this I am no different from other mothers, made it difficult for me to see her objectively at any point in time. How easy it is for a stranger to say of a child, "This child is spoilt and throws tantrums," "This child is cooperative," "This child is bright," "This child is retarded." Easy because a stranger meets the child on a given occasion and forms an overall impression—an impression that may be valid but is one dimensional.

The mother, knowing every stage that has contributed to the present entity, sees at once the present, past, and hopeful future and, in genuine confusion, replies, "Ah! Do you think so? Well, but, you see . . . ." Like the seasoned hunter, she cannot see the forest for the trees; she knows by touch each contour of the land but has no aerial view.

To me, it did not matter that from an aerial view the parts of Melanie's personal jigsaw puzzle did not integrate to form an impressive overall picture. What I knew was each part, by detail of color, shape, and texture. What the objective observers seemed to be looking for was the overall impression—the gestalt presented by Melanie's ill-fitting and poorly coordinated parts.

They observed, for example, that her comprehension of language appeared to be way ahead of all other areas of her development. Indeed, they made a point of commenting on this incongruity between her receptive language and her overall functioning. But they simply could not accept that such a mismatch could be true and attributed her comprehension to intensive repetitive drill on my part and consequent rote learning by Melanie. By *rote learning,* they meant learning that can only be applied within the narrow limits in which the lesson took place. In rote learning, there is no ability to transfer knowledge or apply it in new situations because it is learning that is mechanical rather than creative in nature, and is largely limited to the context in which it was first acquired. According to this view, Melanie's comprehension of language was, in the psychologist's words, a not very meaningful "splinter development."

What effect did this devastating judgment by these professionals have upon me and my view of Melanie?

I wish I could say that their words were only barely influential, that I knew I could retain my own opinion in spite of theirs. But I cannot. In spite of my own experience and observations, I was vastly influenced and depressed by these pronouncements. I think, in the long run, after my initial shock and astonishment, I gradually worked my way to a feeling something like this: I was not convinced that they were right that Melanie had so little potential for intellectual development. But I decided to face the fact that obviously she *functioned* as someone with severe disabilities regardless of what potential she might possess; and after all, how can one consider or describe potential in isolation from a person's performance? The fact was she performed at the level of a person with severe developmental disabilities.

But the corollary to this of course would be, what then? Should I alter my expectations and thus, probably, my efforts and objectives to be more in tune with this terrible diagnosis? I believe that I could not help altering my expectations to some extent. I pride myself on being a realist who manages to cope reasonably well with crises because I take care to prepare myself by accepting whatever appears to be factual. I think I have considerable faith in my own judgment under normal circumstances, but I also have great respect for experience and training. It would have been very difficult for me to maintain my optimism without some encouragement from professional quarters.

Fortunately, I did receive *some* encouragement. Sarah, Melanie's most admiring therapist, was convinced that her colleagues were wrong. She insisted, with no reservations, that Melanie behaved like an intelligent child severely affected by athetoid cerebral palsy, affecting all her muscular coordination including facial expression and speech. She lectured me severely on allowing myself to be influenced in my approach and insisted that I must aim as high as possible for Melanie and at all times expect comprehension. She reminded me of Dr. Karen Pape's explanation of how difficult it would be for whatever intelligence Melanie might have to break through the barriers of severe brain stem and cerebellar damage, and we regretted that Dr. Pape was away in England at that time.

Like Dr. Challenor and my friend Pat at Blythedale Hospital the year before, Sarah recommended Bobath physical therapy as the most important treatment for Melanie, an approach in which a child is repeatedly put through all the normal developmental patterns of movement in the correct sequence in an attempt to diminish the abnormal reflexes of the child with cerebral palsy and to teach the child to exercise conscious control over her muscles. I doubted very much that I would find such a therapist in Trinidad but was determined to continue practicing what principles I had already learned from the OCCC staff and from Sarah.

I have said that I was depressed and discouraged by the assessment that June. Yet I knew that I could never choose to do less than my best for Melanie. Her welfare and development had become the object of my life, and my own satisfaction and sense of personal well-being were now inextricably bound to hers. If I could work successfully with her, accepting her limitations but providing every possible opportunity for her development, then I would be successful in my own eyes and could live happily with myself and with her.

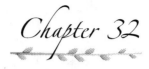

JOAN AND WENDY

I returned home that summer with a plan that had been conceived within months of Melanie's birth and that had been maturing steadily over the 3 years that followed. Melanie would be 3 in September and Mark almost a year. The time seemed right for me to put the plan into action.

I decided to start with a small playgroup in my house for perhaps four preschool children with disabilities. Without any formal training in special education, I thought I could adapt my knowledge of general educational principles, my experience with Melanie, and my volunteer work in Canada. I would learn on the job and, at the very least, would be providing activity and social interaction for the children.

I began by contacting a few doctors and passing around a little card describing the aims of the proposed playgroup. I thought it would probably take a couple of months to get people interested, and that was fine as I would not start before September. Meanwhile, I had agreed to teach a course in an adult education program at the local university for the summer, although I had no idea who I would find to care for the children!

Luck was with me. First of all, my fulfillment of the university commitment was made possible by the unexpected suggestion by my friend Shirley that her 17-year-old stepson, Gerard, who had just left school, should take on my babysitting as a summer job. Accepting this idea required a great leap of imagination for me, since I had assumed the job would have to be done by someone experienced *and* female! But Shirley was confident of Gerard's competence and reliability with children, and I was greatly impressed with this young man who, as the fourth child in a family of eight, had been raised single-handedly by his father after the birth of the last child.

The course I was teaching required my presence 3 days a week, no more than 5 hours' absence from home at a time, and I decided to take the leap. I knew I needed the change and the stimulation of working with adults and decided simply to have faith in Gerard.

Meanwhile, I was receiving one or two inquiries about the proposed playgroup and, by August, actually had one little girl, Raquel, definitely enrolled. I would have been satisfied if I got one or two more by September. But I was not to be left alone with my simple plan. There were grander designs in store for me, and looking back I can hardly believe how easily and naturally the pieces of an unbelievable jigsaw gradually fell into place for me and Melanie.

One night I phoned Dr. Michael Camps, a pediatrician who had promised if possible to refer some children to me. He started off by saying that he had no children to refer but had met a couple of women who had expressed great interest in my idea. One was a speech therapist and one a physical therapist; the latter, he believed, had had some extra training in physical therapy for children with cerebral palsy.

As it turned out, Joan Knowles was a Bobath therapist trained in England by the famous Vera Bobath herself! I could hardly catch my breath when she confirmed this on the telephone, and I accepted her ready invitation to come and discuss my plans with the speech therapist and herself.

The next morning found me at a small house in Woodbrook, a residential and commercial suburb of Port of Spain. I did not know then how central a role this little corner of Trinidad would play in our lives, Melanie's and mine.

Joan Knowles and Wendy Gomez had established together a small clinic offering speech and physical therapy to patients of any age or condition but had a particular interest in children. They were working with two or three children with brain damage whom they felt would profit from an educational program. They were all preschoolers, and there was, up to that time, no systematic program of educational stimulation for this age group at any of the schools for children with disabilities. What these kids needed now was a teacher.

Joan and Wendy's question to me was, "Would you like to join us?"

Would I like to join them? As simple and beautiful as that.

I would like to join them. I *would* join them. I *did* join them and watched incredulously as my little dream of a playgroup for Melanie leaped with one giant step into reality.

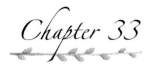

THE SHADE OF
THE IMMORTELLE

Every Trinidadian knows the immortelle tree. In Jamaica it is known as *flame of the forest*. Cousin to the poinciana (called *flambouyant* in Trinidad) and the poui, the immortelle shares the characteristic brilliant bloom of these magnificent tropical flowering trees.

But in Trinidad, the immortelle carries a further specific reputation. Growing tall and wild in the forests, its spreading branches provide shade for the delicate cocoa plant, once a staple crop of Trinidad. The cocoa plant is overly sensitive to direct sunlight, and where the immortelle grows, the cocoa thrives. We called our little school the Immortelle Center for Handicapped Children, and on her 3rd birthday, Melanie had a school to go to.

What can I say of these early beginnings that will not condense them beyond recognition? The school program was offered on a half-day basis until noon, leaving Joan and Wendy to pursue their private appointments in the afternoons and me to return home and relieve my half-day household helper of her responsibility for Mark.

But each half-day's work seemed worth a week's effort, and in no time we all knew that we had embarked upon a challenging but exhausting and frustrating task. For 12 children to begin with, we had what should have been lots of staff, the three of us, plus Gerard, whose handling of Melanie in the summer had been so superb that I knew he would make an excellent assistant. We also had the help of another physical therapist, Deidre, who was recently qualified and so far unemployed, and who gave fully of her time and energy every day on a voluntary basis until the second term, when we were able to give her some monthly pocket money in exchange for her efforts.

Five of us working with twelve children—and still it was not enough! Naturally, the children required intensive attention and training in the three basic areas we worked on; that is, speech and language, motor skills, and cognitive development. The programs and activities were carefully planned and structured, trying to cater to all the individual needs while working within the constraints of the groups. But perhaps the greatest difficulty was the wide mixture of disabilities represented by the children who had come to us, for we literally accepted anyone who came.

By January, the group included five children with cerebral palsy and varying intellectual levels; two children with Down syndrome, one of whom had a hearing impairment; two children with severe hyperactivity and serious language disorders; one girl of 14 with mild retardation, one girl with moderate retardation and hyperactivity; and two boys with severe-to-profound intellectual disabilities, both able to walk independently. Of this entire group, about half were fully toilet trained, and the ages ranged from 3 to 14!

We worked with this group for two terms, assisted further in the second term by another unemployed voluntary physical therapist named Cheryl and by one or two mothers who volunteered on a somewhat uncertain schedule. We were off to a wonderful but terrifying start, and our successes and frustrations were too many and too diverse to catalogue here.

But my concern in the record is Melanie, and I will speak in some detail of her early progress at the Immortelle Center.

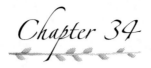

BOBATH THERAPY

Melanie's greatest progress in that time was, to my surprise, in motor development. Joan's progress report in October, after a month and a half of work, described the exercises being worked on and said that "Melanie resists a lot and must be made to do these exercises." But in December, her report began:

> We are very happy to note that for the past month Melanie has really enjoyed her physiotherapy sessions. Consequently she has been very cooperative and is really trying to do the exercises that are expected of her. During our sessions, she now seeks attention from the physiotherapists and is not so eager to roll away and find Mummy.

The last comment reflects a comical feature of Melanie's behavior in the first weeks of school. At first, she spent an awful lot of her physical therapy time rolling across the room to each of the doors to the adjoining rooms, quarreling all the time. As soon as she learned which door led to my room, her intention became quite clear, and she would roll directly up to my door and push her feet against it. But by Christmas, she was rolling up to the therapist instead and tapping on her back with legs or hands.

Her head control and sitting balance improved steadily, but the most exciting development was watching her gradually learn to get up to sitting from lying in exactly the manner she had been taught daily by Joan. She would turn on her side, press both hands on the floor, and push up slowly, legs tucked to

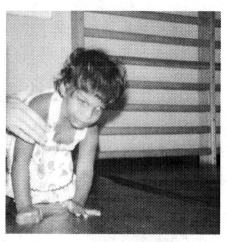

Age 3^1/$_2$, Bobath therapy

one side. She learned this procedure in stages and, for many weeks, could go no further than this first extension of her arms would allow, since if she moved one arm to straighten up more, she would simply lose her balance.

But I remember well the day at the home of our friends Lawrence and Cecile, when I had left Melanie on the bed surrounded by cushions and returned just in time to see her sitting upright, looking intently at the cushions and obviously contemplating what her next move should be. My heart leapt with gratitude.

Another significant moment for us all was the day I heard cheers from the physical therapy room and shouts of "Beth, come!" I rushed in to see Melanie struggling to get up on all fours—she had made it up once by herself and was on her second try. Soon this became a regular feature of her daily voluntary practice, up and down from all fours with no prompting or encouragement whatever.

Indeed, by April, Joan's report described all her progress in motor development and concluded that: "In physical activity Melanie is very highly motivated. She cooperates very well in

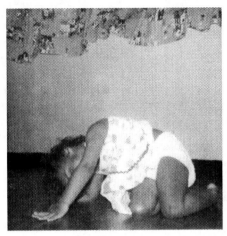

Practicing on her own

physiotherapy sessions and we have noted that she will practice and persevere repeatedly on a physical exercise alone during the day when left unattended."

Melanie was much less consistent and co-operative in speech therapy. Wendy's approach emphasized her receptive language, which I had known to be her strength, and she did make progress in expanding her receptive vocabulary. But she cooperated only when she wanted to, as for example in being taught to differentiate between the primary colors. This required her to point to or touch the correct object when asked for a color. She surprised Wendy by appearing to learn this quite quickly, and in her December report Wendy described her as having already "learned the four basic colors receptively, and has been quite cooperative when doing this task."

However, in January, Melanie would not respond to the color exercise when school reopened, and I have always wondered whether she had forgotten it (a likely occurrence if it was merely a rote response) or whether she really knew the colors so well that she was fed up and refused to do it again. With the advantage of hindsight, I now believe the latter to be the case.

This would always be a puzzling question with Melanie and, I have found, with many children with learning difficulties. I believe that the difficulty here really lies with us as their teachers. Because of our own lack of confidence in their ability, we tend to require many more demons- trations of their knowledge than we would of an ordinary child. We ask the child to perform; he does, and we think, "Well, was that a genuine response or a mistake? Does he *understand* it or has he only learned it by heart?" And so we test him again and

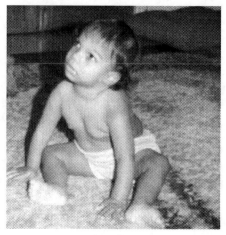

Sitting up!

again, perhaps unreasonably, until the child becomes fed up and starts playing dumb!

Any parent or teacher can readily recognize this behavior in typically developing children of whom we expect so much that we often require only one demonstration to be convinced. I speak very personally on this point because, as a teacher of children with disabilities, I suffered from this dilemma daily basically because my confidence in a child's ability was so unsure.

In any case, Melanie understood more and more of what was said to her and, wonder of wonders, was beginning to point to whatever she wanted instead of just quarreling. Now she would look, point, *and* quarrel. She was becoming quite a character, and everyone who worked with her considered Melanie alert and aware and certainly self-willed and choosy about what she wanted to cooperate with.

We arranged the program so that I was not scheduled to work with Melanie at all, and it was a delight to see Melanie develop her own relationships with several people other than Mummy and Daddy over those months.

The Immortelle Center was the beginning of Melanie's growth as a social being in the sense of interacting in a variety of ways with a variety of people. Come April, she would embark upon a program of further socialization and widening experience, not through my own choice, but in response to circumstances imposed unexpectedly upon our family.

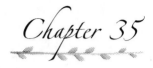
A TEMPORARY GOODBYE

I reacted with despair one day in mid-February when Clive came home with news that he was being asked to leave almost immediately for a 4-month assignment in Toronto! How would I survive 4 months on my own with my two demanding and still totally dependent children?

True, my mother was with me. My father had passed away in the previous August, and our family had flown to Jamaica to say our final farewell to the person I have always considered to have been the most influential figure in my life. I grieved to think how fully he would have shared with us in loving and helping Melanie if only he had been able.

Now Mummy had come to stay with us for a while, still exhausted and coping with her own grief, but always involved and supportive and with a particular passion for Melanie. It was only her presence that made it at all possible for me to consider coping without Clive, but by the end of a month, I knew that 3 more months would be impossible. Mark still woke every night at least once, while Melanie gave her greeting cry between 4:45 and 5:00 a.m. without fail and simply would not shut up until she had been picked up and fed. Then I worked at school all morning and did the housework in the afternoons, all the time trying to respond with some measure of reason to Melanie's incessant calls for attention and Mark's boisterous, rather overpowering personality.

It was just too much, and Joan and Wendy were genuine in their understanding when I told them I could not last after Easter. This would make 2 months without Clive, and since I had every reason to believe that his stay would turn out to exceed the original 4 months, I felt I had no choice but to join him at the end of that term.

Of course, I was filled with guilt at the prospect of deserting the Immortelle Center, but Cheryl, our volunteer physical therapist, agreed to take my place, and I left her detailed outlines of my objectives and activities for the children.

Melanie, Mark, and I left at Easter. I did not know then that this would be good-bye to the first Immortelle Center.

Chapter 36

"YES!"

Melanie burst into life that spring after terrifying us with a 2-week period of depression. For the first 2 weeks in Toronto, she alternated between sleeping and sobbing. She had never been much of a crier, and I had known this sobbing response to occur only if she was in great physical pain. But for 2 weeks, she would burst into sobs every time a new person came into the apartment, and she would sleep until 8 o'clock in the morning and then again for hours at a time during the day. She had no fever and no signs of illness whatever. I soon realized that she was simply heartbroken at being removed from the comforting but growth-inducing shade of our Immortelle.

But it was springtime, and Melanie's temporary withdrawal soon gave way to what seemed an incredible explosion of life and regeneration. It was as if 6 months of intensive daily therapy and stimulation and what had seemed to be gradual development suddenly clicked into place, giving birth to new skills and development in all areas.

The weekend before we left Trinidad, I had seen Melanie sit independently watching television and listening for a full half hour. Within 3 weeks of settling into our beautiful apartment at Toronto's Harbour Front, I discovered that she could bear her weight well enough to stand by herself, leaning her pelvis against the couch and keeping herself upright with outstretched arms. This discovery provided her with tremendous satisfaction, and she loved to be put to stand like this, relaxing her arms and resting her torso on the couch whenever she tired, and then straightening up again.

Very soon I realized that Melanie, when placed on the couch to sit or lie, would turn onto her tummy, stretch her legs out, and quarrel loudly. She wanted to learn to get down to the floor! In no time, with lots of instructions and her own repeated spontaneous practice, she could get her feet down to the floor and assume her standing position. She could not yet get back up, but for months she tried very hard, moving her right knee up to the seat in an effort to propel herself up; however, she simply was not tall enough or strong enough to make that little leap.

The other dramatic development within a month of our move was a sudden leap in her comprehension of language. All at once, I realized that Melanie could now respond to a fairly complex two-part instruction, especially when accompanied by a clear incentive.

The love of her life was music and stories—and what joy I felt to find that I could say to her, "If you want to hear your music, climb down and go over to the record player." She would immediately begin her struggle to get off the couch into her standing position, bend both knees and collapse onto the floor, roll across the room directly to the music, then sit up, point to the records, and quarrel until I made a move to fulfill my promise.

Or at storytime I could say, "Melanie, find the nursery-rhyme book, and I'll read for you," and watch her search the room with head and eyes, then roll off toward the low shelf or table, and try with all her awkward might to pull down this favorite book. She could not hold it but would drag at it until it fell. At this, she would give a huge smile and a squeal and turn to me in delighted expectation.

Her social awareness and interaction had also taken a huge step—she was now very aware of other children and could be quite competitive and persistent in her bids for attention. I believe that one of the happiest occasions of my life with Melanie was watching her engage in what turned out to be a little quarrel with a visiting friend. Garth, Georgia's son, was then 6, and his mother and I chatted as the two children sat on the floor watching *Sesame Street.* Melanie had recently developed a passion for this show and would watch it for the full hour, complaining loudly whenever the adult cast were talking but sitting in rapt attention to all the antics of the Muppets. Her favorite was Kermit the Frog, whose appearance she always greeted with a loud squeal.

On this occasion, it was clear that she wanted to sit beside or, if possible, on top of Garth while watching the show! This grown-up 6-year-old, of course, was irritated rather than flattered by her persistent attention, and Georgia and I watched in amusement as he kept moving his position, only to be relentlessly pursued and leaned upon by an annoying little girl. He kept appealing to his mother, who told him to discuss it with Melanie; so the hour was spent with Garth moving around and offering Melanie repeated reprimands while she, answering in her best quarreling tone, simply rolled after him.

What really turned my heart over on that morning was the sight of Melanie being treated to the normal impatience of a 6-year-old boy! To Garth, she was simply an annoying little girl who was trying quite unreasonably to move in on his territory in front of the television screen. And she, like any 3-year-old-girl, continued to provoke him quite out of patience!

By early summer, one more enormously important development had taken place. I had long been holding her head and forcing it up and down to indicate yes. One day, I asked my little girl if she wanted something to eat, and as she slowly forced her head down, chin to chest, her delighted squeal told me all I needed to know about her.

The rewards were coming thick and fast, and my confidence in Melanie was growing every day.

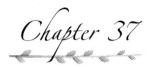

BACK TO SCHOOL

By summer, I knew that what had seemed disastrous luck in February was being transformed into a precious time of opportunity and growth for my whole family. The term of Clive's appointment as manager of the IDC office in Toronto seemed more and more indefinite, but despite the annoying uncertainty, the post was providing him with invaluable experience. It was obvious he would not return in July as expected, and in the face of no fixed plan I decided to take by the horns any bull in sight!

By the time Melanie had emerged from her initial 2-week depression, I had already enrolled her in a half-day program at Centennial Nursery where I had worked as a volunteer 2 years before. This amounted to about 6 weeks of daily stimulation and activity for Melanie and above all the incredible new experience of waving bye-bye to Mummy at the door and going off to school in a taxi provided by the publicly funded program at the OCCC. For Mark, this meant having Mummy entirely to himself for the first time for a few hours a day, and our relationship really bloomed in that time.

For me, it meant beginning to let go of Melanie, beginning to loosen the cord of need and dependence that had bound us so closely together for 3½ years. Of course, I had taken many small steps in that time, from the early days of Mrs. Marshall's and Barb's twice-a-week babysitting, to Gerard the previous summer, and of course, separating her program entirely from mine at the Immortelle Center. But seeing her go off on her own to nursery school was the turning point, and I was grateful for the realization that my experience of being mother to Melanie was becoming more and more normal every day.

Sending my little girl off to school on her own was my first big step that spring. The next was enrolling myself in a couple of special education summer courses at York University on the outskirts of the city. I felt sure we would be in Toronto for the whole summer and saw that I had nothing to lose by this move.

But from the start the hope in the back of my mind was that we might actually be there until about December, by which time I would have enrolled full-time in the diploma in special education course for the winter session and might be able to persuade the faculty to allow me to complete the work in correspondence from Trinidad. In any case, I planned do the summer courses and, if necessary, could always return in subsequent summers to do more.

Our efforts at the Immortelle Center had brought home to me my own need for training in this new field. The challenge had really become harder and harder for all members of our hopeful team, and there were some children, particularly the hyperactive ones, that I absolutely did not know what to do with. I was determined that the Immortelle Center should continue and knew that I, for one, could not succeed in the effort without some formal training.

My motivation was heightened dramatically on the day I received a long letter from Joan describing many discouraging events that had taken place since my departure and saying that Wendy and she found the project really quite impracticable and too frustrating to continue. They would close the school at the end of June and make no move to reopen it until I returned and decided whatever I might like to do.

I read the letter with a sinking heart but no great surprise. We had made a great effort but had, I think, bitten off more than we could chew at that time. Both Joan and Wendy were trained in specific therapeutic disciplines and were excellent at their work. If I had been adequately prepared, I could have run an overall school program with the therapists participating only within the limits of their special fields. But as it was, we were all being required to perform a number of functions for which we were ill-prepared. It was just too exhausting, and splitting 12 fees among five people did not provide an amount that could be considered even minimal remuneration. So I knew what I had to do with whatever time I might have in Toronto and set about putting all the pieces in place.

Melanie spent the summer in a day camp called the Spring Garden Summer Recreation Project for Multiply Handicapped Children. She went off in her taxi every morning and returned in the afternoon covered in paint or sand or some other exciting substance. Simone, Clive's 16-year-old niece, babysat Mark as her summer job, and our wonderful location on the lakefront made it a fun time for them both.

My trip from the harborfront to the northwestern end of the subway line, followed by a bus ride to the campus, allowed me about an hour and a half of reading time daily, and I also had a couple of hours in between classes some days. I was doing a course in teaching the *"trainable retarded"* (a term no longer considered acceptable), which was directly related to my work at the Immortelle Center. The other course was an amazing choice for me but related to my weakest area as a teacher, the function of art in teaching children with special needs.

My studies were exciting, and the feeling of doing something entirely for myself was wonderful. I had not been a student since my master's work in 1973 and I delighted in the irresponsibility of the role of student as opposed to teacher. Of course, I put a great deal into all the activities and am by nature a kind of compulsive participator in any group situation, but still I enjoyed being at the receiving rather than the giving end of the classroom.

It was a full and rewarding summer, and by the end of August, I knew that I would be enrolling as a full-time student in the fall even if I had to leave halfway through the semester.

Chapter 38

MAGNIFICENT HELPERS

Melanie was blessed with a number of magnificent helpers throughout her life. I do not know if they were primarily my helpers and hers by extension or the other way around. But whatever the nature of the relationship, each one of these people provided the unit of me-and-Melanie with specific kinds of support at crucial points in time.

At all times there were my relationships with friends and relatives, all but one of which had proved their incredible strength and value over the years since Melanie's birth. I say all but one because I had one friend who, in our first year in Toronto, met Melanie once and could not face her or me a second time. This person, one of my closest companions in my college days, simply did not have, as we say in the Caribbean, the belly (guts) to face such a flawed child.

But I want to speak here of certain people, most of whom were not necessarily friends, or not initially so, but who came into contact with Melanie and me in their professional capacities, and who, because of the quality of their interest and effort, had a profound influence both on her development and on my confidence in her and in myself.

The first of these people was Venus Mark, the chief midwife at the maternity clinic, who gave me confidence in my ability to care for the most vulnerable of infants, one who could not eat. In our first stay in Toronto, it was Danny and Marg, the OCCC therapists, who provided me with impeccable models of positive and encouraging handling of a not-very-promising baby. Mrs. Marshall and Barb, her first babysitters, showed me that I did not have to be the only person who could care for my delicate child.

At the Immortelle Center, Joan, Wendy, and Deidre had provided Melanie, in 6 short months, with skills that combined to build the bridge from a largely passive to an active existence, and Gerard, in his youthful playfulness, had filled her days with fun and laughter. Shirley, meanwhile, had forced me to seek independence for Melanie at every opportunity. And from our earliest days with her in Toronto, Sara Blacha taught me to believe in Melanie. Vastly impressed with Melanie's progress in gross motor and socialization skills, Sarah was now more than ever convinced of Melanie's potential for development and started weekly therapy sessions with her. Our therapists in Trinidad had pointed out that Melanie chose whether or not to be cooperative. Sarah went one step further in describing my innocent little girl as quite manipulative. Sarah felt that in general I was rather soft on Melanie and allowed myself to be manipulated by her responses. Her approach in therapy was to offer Melanie specific rewards contingent upon her cooperation and really refuse the rewards if Melanie had not worked hard enough. Sarah tried to show me how I could use this technique in everyday requirements at home, such as potty training, self-feeding, and self-help skills in general.

As I watched Sarah work with Melanie, I realized, in great surprise, how low my own expectations and demands were by comparison. Sarah would ask her a question or give an instruction and simply *assume* that she had understood. Further, she routinely accepted any response Melanie gave as genuine and meaningful. If she seemed not to respond, Sarah would usually assume Melanie was either not interested in the request or was being stubborn.

I, by contrast, could seldom escape the questions, "Did she really understand? Was that response meaningful or just a coincidence?" I think that part of the reason for this was a defense mechanism on my part, preferring to expect too little rather than too much and be disappointed again. I could not forget the tremendous contrast between the way I saw Melanie in June 1978 and the devastating opinion of the OCCC assessors. That experience had impressed deeply in me a sense of doubt regarding my own view of Melanie, and now it was Sarah, who handled dozens of children with cerebral palsy weekly, who was insisting that I should expect more.

The extent of Sarah's confidence in Melanie's comprehension and the amount of cooperation she was able to get from her was revealed when Sarah arranged for Melanie to participate in a couple of Sarah's demonstration lectures to student therapists at the local university. Imagine Melanie as a demonstration student!

And it worked! Melanie's level of response and cooperation in both the sessions proved Sarah's lecture point very nicely; that is, not to judge a book by its cover! The students were obviously taken aback at the extent of Melanie's comprehension of all Sarah's requests and instructions and her willingness to try a wide variety of motor tasks, many of which were quite difficult for her.

And so it was that in certain quarters my Little Bird came to be quite a star. And to my great satisfaction, in the next two terms, she was to become a great favorite in her new school.

One of the surprises of that summer was walking into my first class and discovering that one of the lecturers was Martha Carr, the teacher in the developmental class at OCCC in which I had worked as a volunteer 2 years before.

It was great to see Martha again, and through her I was able to find out quickly what avenues were available for school placement for Melanie in the coming term. Martha felt that from my description of Melanie she would be considered appropriate for the developmental level, the lowest-level placement serving

4- or 5-year-olds with multiple disabilities. In spite of her surprising language comprehension, Melanie's lack of self-help skills, such as toileting, self-feeding, walking, and hand skills, made her a totally dependent child, and she would continue to need the intensive attention and stimulation provided by a program such as Martha's.

But Martha's program was really run by the Metropolitan Toronto School Board, responsible for students classified as *"trainable retarded"* and was placed at OCCC because of the health needs and possible medical attention required by many youngsters with multiple disabilities. All applications for placement had to go through this board.

Martha pointed out to me another nice coincidence—that the person in charge of such placement was the senior lecturer in the same course I was taking. My initial application for Melanie to be placed in the program was offered verbally over a glass of draft beer between classes and followed by the appropriate formal letter.

Melanie would be 4 years old that September, of age for the program, and our family would be eligible for this fully state-supported service because Clive, as an employee of the Trinidad and Tobago government, was on a courtesy visa for the duration of his appointment. No problem! Melanie had only to be seen by the board's placement officers so that the appropriate recommendation could be made.

Before I knew it, arrangements had been made for this appointment, and I was putting Melanie through her paces for the assessment by three interested and obviously kindly disposed people who came to our home to do the assessment. Melanie showed herself off to advantage, and as I listened to the observers' comments, I noted that they considered her to be functioning *highly trainable*; that is to say, possibly bordering between *trainable* and *educable* or, in other terminology, between moderate and mild retardation. However, because of her physical disability and very dependent level of functioning, they considered that the best placement initially would be at the developmental level.

I was by then very familiar with the terminology of the field and becoming sensitive to the potential disadvantages of labeling children, having myself been profoundly affected by hearing the label *severely retarded* applied to my child. But I was nevertheless pleased to see that these experienced people did note the disparity between Melanie's comprehension and her overall functional level and appeared to accept it as a reflection of motor rather than cognitive limitations.

The important thing about the question of placement was that she would receive a program appropriate to her needs and be in the hands of competent and caring people. Martha Carr was such a person, and I was greatly relieved to learn that Melanie would be placed in her program. Martha was to become another of the very special people who touched Melanie's life.

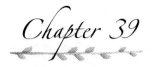

Chapter 39

A HAPPY 4-YEAR-OLD

When I left Toronto in January 1977 with a vomiting baby and a handful of feeding tubes, no one could have convinced me that I would be back within two winters, shopping for overcoats and boots for myself, a healthy 4-year-old schoolgirl, and a vociferous toddling boy. Yet here we were, preparing for winter again, buying the minimum in consignment stores in case Clive's appointment should be terminated in December but making plans that looked for all the world as if we would be here until spring.

I was a full-time student in a graduate diploma course called the Education of Exceptional Students at York University, carrying four courses and having completed two others in the summer program. Most of my classes began shortly before or after noon, leaving me the morning to prepare Melanie for school and spend a couple of hours with Mark. The babysitter, a young woman highly recommended by an agency, would arrive a half hour before the time of my departure and would be in charge until either Clive or I arrived home, depending on the schedule of the day.

The coursework was demanding, but I found that I was not only very motivated but also well prepared by virtue of my previous education and more so by the experience I had gained since

Melanie's birth. I soon realized that what I needed most was skill in setting objectives, breaking a task down into minute steps, and teaching one step at a time. One of the assignments I would have to do was working with a specific child in a special class placement, and this would give me the opportunity to go into

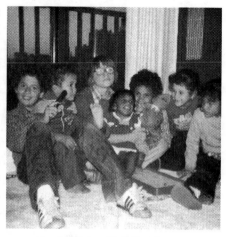

Fourth birthday with Mark and cousins

some depth in this kind of teaching.

Another aspect of the work that was particularly useful for me was visiting and observing a wide variety of special education services and programs in and around Toronto. I saw everything from home-based services to institutional residential programs and began to become aware of the spectrum of possibilities for serving people with disabilities. What amazed me was that all of the services were supported by at least 80% government funding, and I began to realize how ambitious

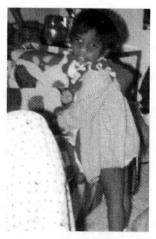

Standing!

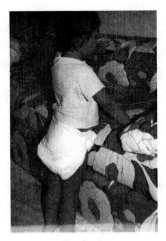

Standing!

and unrealistic our attempt at the Immortelle Center had been to offer specialized services in education, physical therapy, and speech therapy on a totally private basis for one fee. Most programs I saw in Toronto had visiting or consultant therapists, and children would certainly not be seen by these specialists on a daily basis. My course really offered me a widening perspective of the field of special education, and I had no doubt that I would return home prepared to revive the Immortelle Center on a more practicable basis.

All in all, my plans for that fall worked very well, and the

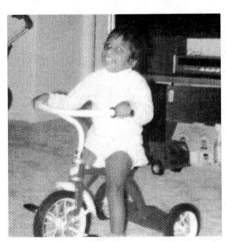

On her bike

babysitter and I were soon crossing paths at the doorway, she taking off her coat as I hurried into mine. Melanie was happy in Martha's little group of four, in which there was a full-time assistant and a volunteer almost every day, as well as a visiting recreational therapist, speech therapist, and psychologist. Melanie soon made her presence felt and was certainly the most advanced in development in the group. With her upright sitting, standing with support, rolling around, and her ability to listen to and understand most of what was said, recognize people by name, and generally make her needs known by vocalizing, pointing, and nodding, she soon began to look

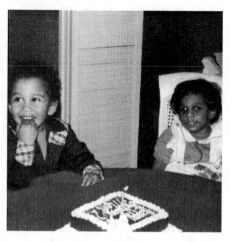

Mark's second birthday

like a star among her more disabled peers.

I remember a visit paid by Martha, Melanie, and me to meet the doctor in charge of the center, in which he expressed delight and surprise at her ability to show, by pointing, who was Martha and who was Mummy. In fact, Melanie was very observant of people and could

identify by name every regular visitor to our house and, on occasion, would surprise us by remembering someone whom she had met only once previously.

I recall Melanie's 4th birthday party that was attended by her five Toronto cousins, about five other children, and of course, all of the adult relatives and some

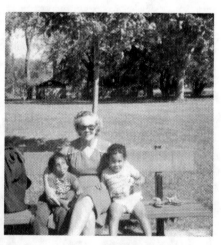

With Mark and Grandma

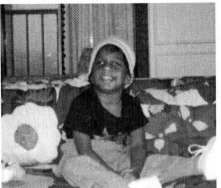

Dressed for school: a happy 4-year-old

friends. Her Aunt Hermia's photographs of the occasion tell all that was important on that memorable day, showing in every shot, an alert, aware, happy 4-year-old in her beautiful red-and-white plaid dress, basking shamelessly in the glory of all the attention being showered on her.

I treasure every photograph of Melanie at every stage of her development because the camera, in its wonderful freezing of a moment, could capture her intelligence and intense receptivity in that moment of stillness before her muscles, in their awkward attempt to communicate, would shatter the image.

Although Melanie's overall coordination was poor, once she had learned a sequence of movement, she could perform it quite smoothly although slowly—such as getting up to sitting from lying, rolling over, or by that Christmas, getting up to standing from kneeling while leaning against a support.

But the movements that were always awkward and discordant in effect were those of head and eyes. When still, she had good head control, but turning her head was such an effort that it often looked as if it might fall off her neck, and the eyes would always go askew. Further, the tendency to a squint, or a drifting eye, had become marked, and the ophthalmologist at Sick Kids' Hospital was recommending surgery to correct it, which would, he said, improve both her depth perception and her looks.

Since we did not know how long we would be in Toronto, Dr. Berry had promised to try to fit her in for surgery whenever an unexpected slot turned up.

Sure enough, in the last week of November, 6 days before my birthday, the hospital phoned to say they would operate in 2 days' time if we were ready. Clive was in Trinidad for a week, and I was scared silly. The thought of my Little Bird in surgery awaking with painful eyes and God knows what else was really awful for me. But I knew we had to use every opportunity available during this unexpectedly productive year. I doubted that in Trinidad the eye specialists would consider it worthwhile improving Melanie's looks given the severity of her disability. I certainly did, so I held my breath and took her into the hospital on the appointed day.

As it turned out, there was one aspect of the surgery that proved problematic, and that was Melanie's unexpected susceptibility to the anesthetic. It was some 6 or 8 hours before she returned to the ward from the resuscitation room, and I was told that the anesthesiologist wanted to speak with me before Melanie's discharge. He made a point of noting the amount and type of anesthetic used, explaining that it was the usual administration for her weight, but that she had taken an unusually long time to come out of it. He advised me to be sure to inform our doctor at home of this if she ever needed surgery again.

Despite this setback, Melanie recovered quickly, coming home the next day as planned, and within a couple of days, her eyes were open and very red and sore looking. I found the look of her eyes quite distressing, but the painkillers prescribed seemed to keep her reasonably comfortable, and by the next week, she was ready for school again. It was a couple of weeks before I could see the difference in her eyes, probably because I found the redness so distracting, but within a week or so her teachers and our friends were commenting on the dramatic difference.

The surgery had not altered her ability to get her eyes where she wanted them to be, but it had certainly ensured that when they got there, they were coordinated instead of one this way and one the other. Now we could tell for sure who or what Melanie was looking at, and I considered this delightful change our best Christmas present that year.

Chapter 40

A NEW DECADE

J anuary 1, 1980, found us still in Toronto. I entered the new decade with an increasing awareness of how well the various pieces of our experience with Melanie were gradually integrating to create a picture of harmony and fulfillment rather than the image of disintegration and failure that had haunted me in the early months of her life. It was like a jigsaw of circumstances and effort in which each separately conceived piece would unexpectedly find its counterpart—each shape and image complementing the next.

Clive's experience in Toronto and his present job had combined to allow us two long-term stays in a city where opportunity for learning and development overflowed for Melanie and me. I had grasped every opportunity with both hands and had been rewarded 100% every time.

We had completed our first stay with a plan that had succeeded where all else had failed in getting Melanie over the hurdle presented by her inadequate feeding system. On returning to Trinidad, my efforts to establish a school for Melanie had resulted in my meeting with therapists whose intervention thrust Melanie into a period of rapid growth and development and planted the seed of a service for others that would grow and flower in years to come. And now, our second stay in Toronto was providing me with the qualification and preparation necessary to develop a career in working with children with disabilities.

Melanie, meanwhile, had graduated to a full-day placement in Martha's class, and Mark was enjoying his three mornings a week in a playgroup, in which his favorite activity was riding on a sturdy three-wheel tractor. This outing allowed him a degree of freedom of movement not available in our apartment.

Clive's appointment was still uncertain—almost on a month-to-month basis, which was annoying and inconvenient for him. But I was convinced that we would be there until April, allowing time for me to complete my course. My intuition proved correct, and it was not until early May that we would finally return home to Trinidad.

But the highlight of our last 2 months in Toronto was the increasing affirmation by professional people of my own early evaluation of Melanie's potential, and I will focus on three very different assessment approaches from which we benefited.

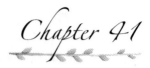

DYNAMIC REASSESSMENT

It was nearly spring again, and Martha had suggested having a formal psychological assessment of Melanie done at the center. I agreed readily, stipulating only that it should not be done by the same psychologist who had canned her so totally 2 years earlier.

Of course Melanie was at much more of an advantage this time, since the psychologist was able to visit her class on a number of occasions, observing her in a variety of situations as well as evaluating her in a formal one-to-one sitting. In this way, she was hoping to give me the scores obtained by Melanie on a standardized test as well as her own impressions outside of the test.

After several interviews with Melanie, the psychologist shared her impressions with me. Until then, I knew little about psychological testing but was beginning to become aware of the limitations of such tests, especially for children with complex or mixed disabilities. Melanie's lack of manipulative skills made it impossible to apply many parts of a test to her, and the psychologist explained that because of this she could not come up with an overall evaluation but would simply describe her level of performance on those areas that Melanie could do.

Basically, this left her with an evaluation of Melanie's developmental level in language, both receptive and expressive. Obviously, the absence of any speech whatever would leave

Melanie with a very low score, and if the absence of speech was a result of motor disability, then once more any overall statement would be inaccurate.

In the long run, all the psychologist was able to give on the basis of her objective data was a description of Melanie's receptive developmental level in language, but that was enough for me. All I really wanted out of this assessment was some reassurance that Melanie's apparent comprehension was recognizable by others and was not merely a figment of the imaginations of those of us who knew and loved her.

And I got that reassurance. The psychologist estimated Melanie's level of language comprehension at about the 2-year-old level, which at just over 4 years of age would place her in the range of moderate retardation. This was not what I would have liked to hear, but I considered it an honest appraisal and assumed that this was, at the very least, the bottom line! I am not ashamed to say that above all this assessment pleased me mainly because it meant that Melanie's record at the OCCC would now reflect an assessment significantly better than the last one!

This was the most conservative of Melanie's three assessments that spring, and I felt that the conventional approach to psychological assessment had been applied in a fair and realistic manner despite its limitations.

At the other extreme was an exciting and unusual 2 days spent with another psychologist recommended to me by one of my professors at York University. Nechama Baum was an Israeli woman of vibrant personality and red hair to match. She was at the time studying the work of Reuven Feuerstein, a German psychologist who had devised an assessment approach that he called dynamic assessment (Feuerstein, Rand, & Hoffman, 1979).

As the name implies, this approach was intended to assess an individual's ability to learn through actually teaching the person a task and observing his or her approach to the problem and the rate of learning. In this way, one might hope to get away from the likelihood of merely testing memory and previous experience. Since that time, I have become well acquainted with Feurstein's model and have learned of its tremendous usefulness for assessing the skills of individuals whose personal, social, or cultural profiles do not fit normative patterns.

Nechama explained first that Feuerstein's procedures had really been designed for adolescents and emphasized that she was attempting to adapt the principles to a completely different situation and would be playing it by ear and coming to her own judgments. It sounded like fun, and Melanie and I were to spend two mornings in Nechama's home.

All of Melanie's therapists and teachers had commented on her tendency to be stubborn and even manipulative to get things done to suit her. I confess that I had never been fully convinced of this, probably because I found it so difficult to draw the line between what she really could do and what she wanted to do, and I tended to give her disability the benefit of the doubt much of the time. Both Sarah and Martha had insisted that my Little Bird had me wrapped around her little finger, but it was not until that morning that I saw it unequivocally for the first time.

In sum, the morning was a battle of wills between Nechama and her small client, with Mummy having been reduced absolutely to observer status. It was 3 hours of intense personal interaction for Melanie in which she demonstrated the full range of behavior available to a person working out her own interpersonal dynamic with another person. Melanie was attention seeking, downright stubborn, willing, unwilling, annoyed, annoying, pleasing, happy, and overall, 100% a responsive little girl trying her best to get her own way. And all of this revolved around her learning a difficult motor task—getting down and then up the stairs.

It was Melanie's idea in the first place when, having refused Nechama's invitation to roll into the living room, she rolled instead to the top of the carpeted stairs and lay on her tummy, looking intently down to the basement and quarreling loudly. Nechama took the cue immediately saying, "Ah! You want to go down the stairs?" An emphatic nod from Melanie, and they were on their way.

But my dependent little girl expected to be carried down the stairs and expressed great annoyance at being told she would have to go down on her knees. Eventually, she followed Nechama's instruction to lie on her tummy and turn around so that her legs were hanging down onto the first step.

For the first half dozen steps or so, Melanie's new teacher showed her all the movements required, actually moving her limbs for her but gradually giving less and less support. When Melanie first realized that the support was being withdrawn, she simply put her head down on the step and refused to go any further. But this did not last too long, and she soon started stretching or flexing one limb at a time as instructed, her legs being, as usual, much more efficient than her stiff arms, which Nechama supported with the minimum assistance possible.

It was the first time Melanie had tried this task, but she was ready for it, having already learned to get down off the couch. However, I considered it a difficult task because of the steep slope of the stairs; I tried to say so to Nechama but was reminded that I was not allowed to participate!

Their progress down the stairs must have taken half an hour or so, with Melanie alternating between cooperation and refusal. When she finally made it, she was rewarded with great cheers and a bit of cookie. She rolled around the room, exploring for a while, and when she seemed tired of that, Nechama told her she would have to climb with her back up the stairs since the rest of our snack was upstairs.

This was the beginning of the real battle. Melanie tried everything she could think of. She gave her sign for hunger (hand to her mouth), she quarrelled at Nechama, at me, at another lady present, she stretched her arms up to be picked up, she pointed up the stairs, she cried real tears, and finally, in a last bid for power, lay down and closed her eyes, pretending to sleep! But Nechama was adamant and walked up the stairs telling Melanie that we were going for a snack, and when she was ready to climb up, she should call us!

Melanie quarreled until we were out of sight, and then there was silence. I could hardly believe that half an hour went by without a sound from her, and then finally, a loud call in a very annoyed and imperative tone. Nechama went coolly to the top of the stairs, and I doubted my ears as I heard her say, "Well, you're ready to come up are you? That's right, get on your knees, and I'll come and help."

And sure enough, as I peeped around the stairs, there was my little lady struggling up on to her knees, body propped against the low first step and still quarreling loudly. She had given in, but not without a speech.

From there on, the point had been made—that Nechama was in charge and Melanie could choose to cooperate or not. For the most part, she chose to cooperate, and her struggle up those stairs was beautiful to watch. Nechama knew just how much help to give her, and together they made it up the stairs in time for a snack and a few of Melanie's favorite games.

Upon our arrival on the second morning, I put Melanie on the floor, took off her coat, and walked away. She rolled across to the top of the stairs, turned on her tummy, stretching legs behind her down the stairs, looked around at Nechama, and gave a grin and her squeal of delight! In our discussions afterward, Nechama made no attempt to objectify or quantify her impressions. She had worked with Melanie intensively for two mornings and came to a definite impression: Melanie had a mind of her own and had demonstrated fairly typical 4-year-old behavior, culminating in cooperation and learning of the elementary steps of a motor task that was a great challenge to her.

Nechama focused on Melanie's manipulative and resistant behavior and spoke seriously of her need to be curbed of this and to be forced to develop more independence. She continued in this vein, never addressing directly the question I wanted to hear answered—the question of what she thought of Melanie's intellectual capacity. As she continued, I finally managed to express this thought in a sort of apologetic, indirect manner, and Nechama, suddenly recognizing my main concern, responded emphatically, "She is *not* mentally retarded! Of course she is not. Look at the extent of her physical handicap, and look at what she is able to express and learn in spite of it! And she is only 4! Look at my son, and try to imagine what he looked like at 4. He was much worse than her physically and could show almost nothing of what he knew, and look at him now!"

And all of a sudden, I realized that ever since the devastating assessment 2 years before, I had never stopped comparing Melanie to the normal child of her age. That day at Nechama's home, I did look at her 18-year-old son, severely affected by athetoid cerebral palsy and a hearing impairment, and saw a young man who, in spite of his extreme handicap, had learned to walk, however awkward his gait; to talk, however difficult his speech was to understand; to type so that he could clarify his conversation for his listener; and having just completed the requirements for the Grade 12 diploma, had been accepted into a community college in Toronto.

I felt a rush of awe and hope as it finally dawned on me that when I looked at Melanie, I must think not of what a normally developing 4-year-old should look like but of what a 4-year-old with severe cerebral palsy might look like.

And even then, what I did not realize was the real extent and severity of damage that Melanie had suffered. It was Dr. Karen Pape and the incredible machinery of modern medicine that would reveal this in the space of a few weeks.

Chapter 42

CT SCAN

I had first heard of a CT (computed tomography) scan in 1976 when Dr. Pape, puzzled by some of the peculiarities of Melanie's development, had told us a bit about this relatively new piece of medical technology. At that time, she had decided against using this procedure, which I understood to be a sort of X-ray technique for revealing the actual structure and conformation of the brain itself, because she felt that the technology was still too new to be reliable, especially in a baby as small as Melanie was then.

Dr. Pape was back in Toronto in the winter of 1980, and Melanie and I paid her a visit at Sick Kids' Hospital where she had resumed her duties. Once more, Melanie proved a fascinating study for this perceptive doctor. She was struck by the sharp disparity between Melanie's comprehension, which was now demonstrable beyond doubt, and her rather immobile and unexpressive face. Melanie's face really did not reflect her comprehension, and it was her newly acquired skills of pointing, nodding, and appropriate responses of the body that made it clear that she understood both language and her environment in general.

For example, she could by then point out a picture of an item requested besides being able to identify the item itself. In fact, one of my projects of the winter was making a collection of photographs and clippings with which to compile picture boards, which Melanie could use to point to the information she wanted to communicate. So far, we had had the most success with her food picture board from which, for example, she could choose to have a banana rather than an orange instead of having to quarrel unintelligibly through whatever treat Mummy had decided on.

Methods such as this clearly revealed her understanding, and Dr. Pape was becoming more convinced of her original impression of Melanie and wanted to test it objectively. Her feeling was that Melanie had suffered severe brain stem and cerebellar damage but that the cortex (which controls intelligence and some gross motor functions) was probably intact.

She explained that although the functions of the cerebellum were still not properly understood, it was known to affect overall muscle coordination, coordination of eyes and hands, and possibly control of the facial muscles. She referred to another child she had known whose developmental features were similar to Melanie's and whom the CT scan had shown to have suffered severe cerebellar damage with no evidence of damage to the cortex.

Now Dr. Pape was suggesting a CT scan for Melanie, and my first reaction was resistance. What would we gain from knowing the insides of my child's brain? Suppose we learned something terrible and unacceptable! Wouldn't it be better not to know?

But Dr. Pape felt that the scan would reveal considerable information about the nature and extent of brain damage and that whatever we learned would help us to understand and help Melanie better. She expected the scan to yield information that would be helpful and productive, and her optimism and confidence came across so clearly that I could not help being influenced by it.

It was late in April that Dr. Pape came up with this recommendation, and by then we knew that we would be leaving Toronto in mid-May. There was not much time, and Melanie's appointment for the scan was literally squeezed in at the last minute, a week before we were scheduled to leave.

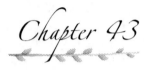

BRAIN GAZING

It was May 9, 1980, and the Radiology Department of Toronto's Hospital for Sick Children felt for all the world like a science-fiction fantasy. There was chrome and Plexiglas everywhere, and the huge structure on which Melanie's 25 small pounds lay could, for all I knew, have been a space machine operated by the invisible but ever-present tentacles of Big Brother.

Certainly it was a room for seeing, brilliantly lit, with no kind of softness or shadow; and behind their sheet of glass, the medical seer-men fixed their gaze on the images projected onto a screen. The images were of Melanie's brain as the revolving eye of the X-ray camera peered, I thought, into her very soul.

No doubt I was the only person in the room who saw it all in this way. What seemed awesome and eerie to me was a matter of day-to-day routine for the others. This procedure was a product purely of man's technology and, as such, could contain nothing superhuman or mysterious.

But it was a mystery to me, as Melanie had been a mystery, and as I stood in the sterile brightness of the room, I was not at all sure I wanted her innermost self elucidated by some omniscient machine.

This was on Friday. Dr. Pape had promised to call me on Monday with the results, and as I struggled through the weekend, I knew that I did, after all, want to know everything possible about

my special Little Bird. On Monday, my hand trembled on the
receiver as I listened to Dr. Pape's calm voice, summarizing their
initial impressions of the CT scan.

"Beth, we have good news and not-so-good news. I'll start
with the good."

As she had expected, the picture showed a small but intact
cortex with no evidence of any lesions. The upper part of Melanie's
brain, then, looked normal though small.

I held my breath, trying to control the leap of gratitude that
I felt in case what would come next should be so terrible as to
negate the wonderful confirmation of the message I had been
receiving from Melanie's eyes ever since her birth. But the news to
come was a dramatic reinforcement of Dr. Pape's theory. She had
been right about the cerebellar damage, but the extent of this was
much more extreme than she had imagined. Where Melanie's
cerebellum should have been, the scanner showed what Dr. Pape
described as two small lumps and a large space. It seemed, she said,
that most of the cerebellum was simply not there.

As I struggled to cope with an overwhelming sense of
incredulity, Dr. Pape continued, explaining that although she felt
this was the most likely explanation of the space, there was also a
slight possibility that it might really be a large cyst covering the
cerebellum. Although unlikely, this possibility should be ruled out
by a further scanning procedure. This would involve injecting fluid
that would flow into the space, or if there should be a cyst, the fluid
would flow around it, outlining it. With a mounting feeling of
unreality, I agreed to the procedure; we were on the verge of a real
understanding of Melanie at last, and there could be no turning back.

As I put down the phone, I knew this conversation would be
one that would have perhaps the greatest impact on me and my
feelings about Melanie. Over the years, I had developed a kind of
empathy with her that had enabled me to anticipate her very
breathing, her choking, her smiling, her swallowing, and her tears.

Sometimes I used to feel as if she had never really left my body, as if she was still an extension of me.

As this new information began to sink in, I was flooded with awe at the knowledge that now I was looking right inside her, looking with knowing eyes into that part of her that should be most unfathomable, most unavailable to me. I felt as if now our symbiosis could be complete; now I could really know her, could really feel for her and with her. And somehow, I felt sure that Dr. Pape's interpretation of what the camera had shown would be correct, that it was indeed a picture of a competent but incomplete brain.

That Thursday, Clive and I waited for Dr. Pape after the examination had been done and tried to absorb all she had to say.

The metrizamide had done its job, filling what was certainly a large space and indicating clearly that there was very little cerebellum to be seen. The two small lumps, she explained, were thought to be atrophic cerebellar hemispheres—in other words, all that was left or all that had developed of the cerebellar portion of Melanie's brain. The brain stem could barely be seen but appeared to be small and underdeveloped.

Of course I was full of questions about the appearance of the cortex. Dr. Pape explained that its being smaller than normal could suggest some amount of mild atrophy but that this was by no means definite. What was most important, she stressed, was that the scan had revealed no signs of damage to this portion of the brain.

While the scan was not perfectly reliable in picking up every detail, the information it had yielded certainly ruled out a diagnosis of overall brain damage and indicated clearly that there was no reason Melanie should not be in possession of good intelligence. So the scan could not prove or demonstrate her level of intelligence, but it could provide no reason to doubt the signs of intelligence she showed.

I had to ask, "But is the scan capable of clearly demonstrating limitations to intelligence?" Dr. Pape's reply was emphatically yes. The scan would certainly show any large lesions—that is, damage that was severe enough to seriously impair intelligence—and this was certainly not the case with Melanie.

Dr. Pape went on to explain that the cerebellar damage would, of course, seriously interfere with her ability to express what she knew because of poor control over the muscles of her face, eyes, arms, and hands and

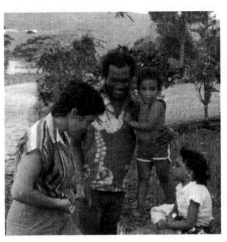

Four and a half, with Mummy, Daddy, and Mark in Jamaica

because of a severely impaired ability to visualize and utilize spatial relationships. Dr. Pape's favorite example of the latter impairment was fascinating. Most people, she pointed out, can pick up a pen and put it in their shirt pocket without having to look at the pocket; they simply know exactly where the pocket is and how to get the pen into it. A person with severe cerebellar damage, such as athetoid cerebral palsy, would have great difficulty accomplishing this apparently simple task. Certainly, I could see this impairment in every move Melanie made.

Dr. Pape now felt certain of her original impression of Melanie. The diagnosis, as far as she was concerned, was clearly one of athetoid cerebral palsy with severe cerebellar damage but, most probably, good intelligence.

I had one last question. I wanted Dr. Pape to negate once and for all the words that had haunted me for 2 years, the words of that devastating diagnosis: "Gross global brain damage with severe mental retardation."

She replied, "The damage is gross, but it is certainly *not* global."

Months later, Dr. Pape reiterated this diagnosis in a letter in which she responded to my continuing hesitation to believe that Melanie's intelligence could be totally normal:

> If you feel better holding on to the idea of abnormality, then I think you just have to put your mind to it that it is at the good end of the spectrum, not the bad end. I think that all the information we have at this point indicates that we should push on with Melanie and expect the best. I don't think her progress is going to be rapid, but I think she has already shown you that slow and steady progress is her way.

With Sarah, Martha, Nechama, and Karen Pape believing in Melanie, I could begin again to trust my own impressions. And what perfect timing, for once more it was time to leave.

In mid-May, we left the cool spring weather for our land of eternal summertime, stopping in Jamaica to visit my brother Philip, who had recently moved there. He had accepted a job as the physician for Reynolds Jamaica Mines, an aluminum mining business that was at the time a huge contributor to Jamaica's economy. Clive, Mark, Melanie, and I spent a few days breathing in the beauty of this idyllic spot, located among the rolling hills of the Parish of St. Ann. We were on our way home.

Chapter 44

MERCEDES AND ELIZABETH

B ack in Trinidad I had one consuming concern—how to reestablish the Immortelle Center. After my exposure to a variety of programs during my course in Toronto, I had begun to develop a clearer idea of how I could adapt what I had learned to our much more circumscribed situation.

First of all, I realized that our ambitious attempt to offer all the necessary therapeutic services under one cover and on totally private funding had been financially impossible. My idea now was to establish a more conventional type of school that I would operate along with some teaching assistants, augmented by speech and physical therapy services on a consultant basis. The latter, I felt, could be engaged by me with a view to helping me incorporate appropriate therapeutic principles into my program planning. This should only cost me, possibly, a couple sessions a month. Beyond this, therapy sessions could be arranged for individual children at a separate cost to be agreed on between the therapist and the parent.

As it turned out, Wendy, who had had her first baby during that year, was now doing speech therapy at home and would not be available for extra work. Regarding the original Immortelle Center, both therapists saw it as a worthwhile experience that neither of them wanted to repeat!

However, Joan was certainly interested in my new idea and was willing to participate. Most important, she was now using only half of the Brabant Street premises and offered me the other half to operate the school. So I had a location for the school and the consultant services of an excellent physical therapist. The next step was to find the pupils.

Of our previous pupils, several had found a place in a small home-based program, and others had left the country for one reason or another. Of that original group, only three, including Melanie, would return to the Immortelle Center. So I had to do some advertising, mainly through the newspapers and through an interview I managed to get on a popular morning television program. I decided that if I got half a dozen pupils, I would start with one assistant and let things emerge from there.

I planned to organize the school into two basic groupings, a nursery section into which I would take very young children regardless of the severity of the disability or the extent of their dependence. In the classroom section I would place older children whose functional level would have to include basic self-help and independence skills and sufficient attention span to allow them to remain seated and attend to preacademic or academic skills.

By early August, I knew I had enough pupils to start and was beginning to realize that the problem would not be simply getting pupils, but getting pupils whose families could afford to pay fees. One way around this would be to try to get sponsorships from business firms or service clubs. By a series of coincidental conversations, I soon got just the introduction I needed to try out this idea and found myself being invited by the local Rotary Club to put my idea to its members at one of their regular luncheons. To my amazement, my talk yielded offers of four sponsorships—one from a businessman in his private capacity, one from a large foundation, and two from the Rotary Club itself.

My luck was holding, and I knew that if I could just find the right two assistants, I could start in September with 10 children. In the summertime, all the young people just out of high school in Trinidad live on tenterhooks awaiting their examination results, making it difficult to get a commitment from

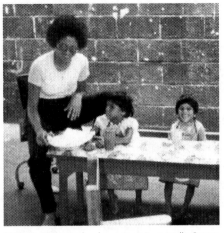

With Mercedes and a classmate at Immortelle Center

any such person before the end of August.

However, Elizabeth, the daughter of one of my dearest friends, Sheila, had indicated an interest in working with me, and I knew that her gentle and thoughtful manner would be well suited to working with children. Exam results notwithstanding, I felt fairly sure that she would in fact take the job, and I wondered where the second person would emerge from.

Gerard, who had worked so well with us in the first year, was no longer available, having secured a job at the School for the Physically Handicapped. He had developed a keen interest in the field and hoped to go on to a teachers' college in the next academic year.

Shirley and Henri, Gerard's parents, had suggested that Mercedes, one of his sisters, might be a good candidate for the position. I had met Mercedes only briefly that summer when, having just left school, she had come with Gerard to babysit Melanie and Mark on a few occasions. She was a lively, outgoing 17-year-old with a wide, infectious smile, boundless energy, and a flair for playing imaginatively with children. Melanie had taken an instant liking to her, responding with delight to her dramatic and very physical approach.

The night after the omnipotent O-Level exam results were published, Mercedes appeared at my door with shy eyes and a smile that stretched from ear to ear, saying, "I've come to apply for the job." As her combined buoyancy and diffidence reached me, I knew that, following the pattern of the previous few years, things were emerging with a rightness and naturalness I could not have planned, and I felt sure that everything would continue to flow from there.

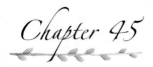

Chapter 45

THE SPREADING BRANCHES
OF THE IMMORTELLE

What grew from there were the spreading branches of the Immortelle as our small effort seemed to take onto itself the color and charisma of its chosen symbol.

In that first term, days at our little center were characterized by the gaiety and energy of my two helpers. Together they exuded all the beauty of youth, the sense of fun and freedom, and the idealism and faith of young people at the brink of adulthood. To them, their charges were simply children, their disabilities incidental, and they approached them with an easy acceptance that allowed neither pity nor condescension.

In addition to Mercedes and Elizabeth, I also had another very valuable helper. Glenna was an experienced special education teacher from Toronto, who, accompanying her husband on a 1-year assignment in Trinidad, had found herself stranded at home in the role of expatriate housewife. Glenna volunteered her services three mornings a week and proved to be the source of innumerable innovations and strategies that it would have taken me years to develop on my own. Her experience and initiative were invaluable to me at that time, and her presence in the classroom made it possible for me to spend time in the nursery group making sure that Mercedes and Elizabeth were on the right track. But this was hardly necessary, as their naturally complementary personalities provided everything I could require, and their sense of duty and responsibility made supervision superfluous.

As the Immortelle Center thrived, so did Melanie come into full bloom with all the attention and activity. In particular, she responded unreservedly as Mercedes invaded her life with movement and laughter, and I watched with joy as the relationship between these two became more reciprocal with every day.

Mercedes teased Melanie endlessly and involved her in all sorts of little games and routines that Melanie delighted in. Soon the sight of Mercedes arriving at our home to babysit was enough to evoke an ear-to-ear smile and Melanie's loudest squeal. Mercedes's babysitting, of course, included Mark, and her talent with children showed also in this relationship.

By November, we were confident enough in Mercedes's ability to handle both children that we were able to take off for Tobago on the weekend of my birthday, leaving her in charge with the additional support of Gerard coming to sleep overnight.

Amidst all of these events, Melanie was becoming quite a character. One of her developments that year was a comical turning of the head for a *no* response. I had worked with her on this by holding her head with both my hands and turning it from side to side, saying "No. This is how you say no." When she finally initiated this on her own, her total turning of the head from extreme left to right and back again looked so strange that it was several occasions before I realized that it was intended to mean "no." My realization of her intent came one day as I was taking her into the shower; as we stepped into the cubicle, I realized that she was writhing from side to side in a very deliberate manner. Pausing, I asked her what was wrong, and leaning back to look at her properly, it suddenly struck me that most of the effort to turn seemed to be focused on her head with her body following involuntarily.

Gasping in surprise, I exclaimed, "What are you saying, Melanie? Are you saying no?" With her wildest squeal of delight, she nodded the most emphatic yes I had ever seen, touching her chin right down to her chest! This was a wonderful addition to her communication system, except that instead of cooperating in the use of her picture board for pointing out what she wanted, my young lady went through a phase of engaging us in a game of 20 Questions: She would turn her head from side to side until we got to what she wanted, at which point she would stop turning her head and start nodding yes instead.

Another key feature that started to emerge was a new level of initiative that often proved highly comical though sometimes potentially dangerous! First, Melanie could now get into trouble by interfering with things! My favorite memory is of the day she wrecked the needle on my friend Sheila's record player. While sitting on the floor listening to one of her favorite songs, it seems Melanie decided to try to change or repeat the record, so she rolled over to the turntable, which was on a low table, and made a swipe at the arm, causing the needle to scrape across the record and break. When I went to pick her up and Sheila told me what had happened, I couldn't contain my delight at the thought that Melanie had actually gotten into trouble! Against Sheila's protests, I insisted on paying her for the needle. What a treat to have to apologize for my little girl's naughtiness!

Another moment was simultaneously hilarious and terrifying. Our quiet suburban cul-de-sac was so safe that, when inside, I habitually left the door not just unlocked but wide open. It was my habit also to putter around the house while Melanie sat on the floor in the living room engrossed in the antics of her favorite television characters. From her days of watching *Sesame Street* in Toronto, her favorite had been Kermit the Frog. Recently though, she had developed what I can only call a crush on Mr. Rogers. So great was her enchantment with the theme song for this show—

"It's a Beautiful Day in Our Neighborhood"—that I could comfortably work in the kitchen or even read a book in the bedroom throughout the entire half hour of this show.

One day, there was a near disaster. I was actually lying in bed, as engrossed in my book as I thought Melanie was in her idol, when I heard a voice calling from the street, "Miss, Miss! The baby! The baby!" Leaping to the window, I saw a young boy standing at our gate pointing to the steps. Melanie was seated on the bottom-most step, almost into the yard, which stood only a couple of feet from the gate. I can find no words to capture the mixture of horror, disbelief, and joy that propelled me from my bedroom to those steps. As I scooped her up into my arms, she beamed the widest smile I had ever seen, squealed the loudest squeal I had ever heard, and wiggled like an excited puppy. It had never occurred to me that Nechama's coaching in turning around and crawling belly-first down the steps would ever have resulted in my Baby Bird trying to run away from home!

At school, Melanie's increasing comprehension and sense of humor were perfect fodder for the youthful imagination of Mercedes and Elizabeth. An occasion that stands out in my memory was one day when the laughter from the kitchen culminated in a shout for my attention. I entered the room to see Melanie perched high on top of a stack of boxes, quarreling loudly at Mercedes and Elizabeth, whose giggles told me they were up to some trick with her. They said, "Beth, we've told her that if she can tell you which one of us put her up there, then we'll take her down! You ask her who did it!"

The girls had positioned themselves far enough away from her and from each other that pointing in either direction would entail considerable effort on her part. In this way, they wanted to ensure that her choice would not be construed as accidental. Obediently, I said, "Melanie, who put you up there?" Putting one hand down to ensure self-support as her body turned, Melanie

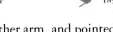

twisted around to face Mercedes, lifted the other arm, and pointed accusingly to the culprit. Her correct answer was greeted with delight from all of us and rewarded by a vigorous spin through the air from her favorite but provoking friend.

By this time, I was using a variety of pictures to find out how much Melanie knew of her environment and how much she understood of language. I was constantly surprised at her responses. We had passed the stage of asking her to identify a picture, that is, simply a labeling response to questions such as, "Show me the house," "Show me the cat," and so forth. I had moved on to questions designed to have her make associations, such as, "Which one says *meow*?" Or to demonstrate knowledge of the functions of objects, such as, "Which one do we drive in? Which one do we hear with?" Melanie would correctly answer a wide variety of such questions upon being asked for the first time.

One of the more complex of such questions involved the rather abstract concept of time, and Melanie's immediate correct response was truly revealing. Showing her four pictures, I asked her to point to the one that showed the time when we go to sleep. She promptly pointed to a picture of nighttime with quiet houses and moon and stars standing out against a dark sky. Similarly, her wide receptive vocabulary could be recognized through a question such as, "Which one tastes delicious?" In response to this, she would choose a picture of cookies.

While her receptive language developed rapidly that year, there were next-to-no new developments in her ability to make sounds. To be precise, she did learn to make one new sound, and this was an absolute charmer!

While rolling one day, she discovered that by pressing her mouth against the floor, she could repeat the sound "du, du, du." She practiced this for weeks and then began to try it while sitting up. I noticed that she would always bend her head down, chin to chest, in order to make this sound, and the reason for this posture soon became evident. In imitating the movement, I discovered that as I put my chin down,

my tongue would move
naturally into place
against my upper palate
just behind my front
teeth, and in this
position, the sound of
"du" was easy to make!
Soon, saying Daddy was
one of Melanie's favorite
activities, and as we
would say, "Melanie, say
Daddy," down would go
her chin, resulting in a
long series of "du du du
dus" followed by a big grin.

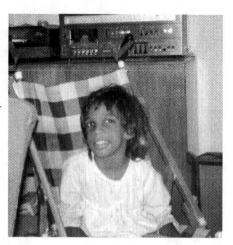

A happy 5-year-old

Despite her limited communication system, Melanie was able
to make herself understood in many important ways. The best
example I can think of was an occasion in which she developed an
ear infection, which I suspected by her fretfulness and constant
rubbing of one ear. I asked her if her ears were hurting, and she
nodded yes, touching the right ear. In the doctor's office, after I
had told him of the problem, he asked me which ear I thought it
was. I turned to Melanie and said, "Which ear is hurting you,
Melanie? Touch it, so we'll know." Without hesitation Melanie
touched the right ear, and sure enough, upon examination, this was
the ear that proved to be inflamed.

Dr. McDowall was delighted at her communication and, as
usual, complimented me on her wonderful progress. I thanked him
and pointed out that no matter how hard I worked with her I could
not elicit from Melanie more than she had within her. By then, I
was sure of Melanie's intelligence and proud that at last she was
able to demonstrate it to other people.

Chapter 46

A FAIRY-TALE MORNING

I t was July 30, 1981, and all the romantics in our part of the hemisphere had set their alarm clocks for 4 o'clock in the morning to witness, via satellite transmission, the royal though ill-fated wedding of the century—Prince Charles and Princess Diana of England.

In our little corner, Melanie could hardly believe her good luck in being picked up by Mercedes the minute she called out at a quarter to 5 and being taken into the living room to watch the television. Her morning routine, after all, usually involved being told, "Good morning, Melanie," and having her tape-recorded music turned on to play for the next three-quarters of an hour while the rest of the household slept until 6 o'clock or, at least, until the sun rose.

But on this unusual morning, here we were—Mercedes, Melanie, and I—glued to the TV screen long before dawn, watching the fairy-tale coaches of the British royalty parade their centuries-old opulence before the world. As we waited for the modern princess to float by, encased in folds of taffeta, her Prince Charming at his royal military best awaiting her, I tried to explain to my little girl that the prince and princess would get married and live happily ever after just like in the stories she so much loved to listen to.

But like that now-famous marriage, the day that started in a fairy tale was to end in a nightmare.

It was the Thursday before the August 1st long weekend, and I had dozens of last-minute details to finalize for our summer camp program at the Immortelle Center, which was to begin the following Tuesday.

Anne-Marie, the new assistant who had joined us after Easter, had offered to run the day camp with the help of Mercedes, Elizabeth, and some volunteers. I had enrolled both Melanie and Mark in the program and was looking forward to 3 glorious weeks of irresponsibility from 9:00 a.m. to 2:00 p.m. every day. In fact, my plan was to use those 3 weeks to bring up to date the documentation of my experience with Melanie. Up to that point, this little chronicle described Melanie's development until about 9 months of age. I had written most of it during my pregnancy with Mark and had never had the time or energy to continue since his birth.

This Thursday and Friday then were to be devoted to finalizing all the preparations for the camp. Mercedes and I would do what we could at school together, and then I would go off on various errands while she kept the children. A young volunteer, Sandra, was coming along for the day to help out and to get accustomed to Melanie, whom she was meeting for the first time. We spent some time at school doing odd jobs and making never-ending lists of what was yet to be bought. The two biggest tasks of the day were how to get the little drive-yourself car fixed and to figure out what additional materials were needed to erect the vinyl wading pool I had bought. I had an idea that instead of going to all the trouble of packing around the pool's circumference with earth, I could probably achieve the necessary stabilizing effect by padding it with foam. However, I was not quite sure of this and decided to run all the other errands first, and then go to the foam factory if I had the time.

I had planned to leave both Mark and Melanie with the girls, but Mark was in a cranky mood, and Mercedes and Sandra had work to do that I did not want him to interfere with. So I decided to take him and leave only Melanie with them.

As I was opening the gate to go, Melanie, standing in her walker in the yard, started to quarrel loudly. Mercedes said, "What, Melanie? What do you want?" As Melanie pointed to the gate, I said, "You want to come?" She nodded a vigorous yes, and I said, "No, sweetheart, Mummy has too much to do; you stay here, I'll be back soon." I blew her a kiss and left.

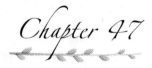

Chapter 47

FROM FAIRY
TALE TO NIGHTMARE

It was afternoon by the time I had finished most of the errands, including a lengthy visit to the foundry where the car was to be fixed. I knew I should go back to school because I had already been away longer than planned and had not even left lunch for Melanie. However, that was a small problem as I knew Mercedes would find something for her to snack on until I got back. If I didn't go to the foam factory, then it would mean a separate trip on the next day just for that. I was, by then, quite annoyed with myself for buying that type of pool, since getting it set up was proving to be such a nuisance.

I got to the foam factory at about 1:00 p.m., and it must have taken half an hour for me to explain to the foreman exactly what I wanted. When we finally had it figured out, he gave instructions for the foam to be cut and suggested that I have a seat, as it would take 10 or 15 minutes.

I thought of phoning school, but on discovering that the phone was upstairs, I decided to leave the call until the foam was ready and I'd be able to tell Mercedes I was on my way. But about 10 minutes later, there was still no sign of foam, and I was beginning to feel uneasy about the lateness of the hour and Mercedes having no real meal for Melanie.

So Mark and I trekked up the little wooden stairs to the office telephone.

I had quite forgotten that Sandra was also at school and did not recognize the voice that answered the phone. For a moment I thought I had the wrong number, but the voice was breathless and trying to tell me something.

Then I realized it was Sandra, but I could not understand what she was saying. I said, "Let me speak to Mercedes." But she kept saying no. Then all of a sudden, the words came through to me, "Mercedes is feeding Melanie, and she is choking." My cheeks tightening, I could hear my own voice giving the instructions like an automaton.

"Sandra, tell her to put Melanie's back against her chest, place a fist under her diaphragm, and pound upward on the fist with the other hand. That will force air up into her throat, and the food will come out."

I repeated these instructions over and over, my heart pounding and my mind reeling. In the past 9 months, Mercedes had fed Melanie as many times as I had and had never had to call on me for help in handling one of Melanie's frequent but relatively simple chokes.

This choke must be different. I could hear the panic in Sandra's soft voice. I knew Mercedes would use her common sense in a crisis, but had I ever taught her this emergency procedure, which had been demonstrated to me in Canada, and which I had to use one terrifying night earlier in that same year?

On that occasion, Melanie had choked suddenly on a piece of raw carrot that Mark had put into her mouth, meaning to share his snack with her. As Clive and I rushed with her in the car to the doctor, it was this procedure that had finally dislodged the carrot. On arriving at Dr. Camp's home, he verified that it was the most effective procedure for choking and demonstrated it again for Clive and myself.

But had I ever taught it to Mercedes? I could remember talking about it with her, but had I ever really demonstrated it and had her practice it? Could I have been so complacent about the improvement in Melanie's feeding?

As these thoughts whirled through my mind, I heard Sandra's voice, "Something's coming up—no, it's only saliva, Mercedes is still trying."

I told her to keep trying while I phoned Clive and the doctor. But Clive's line was out of order. He was 5 minutes away from Melanie, and I could not get him.

I tried Dr. Roache, whose office was next door to Clive's. Also out of order. I phoned school again to hear Sandra's voice repeating, "She's still choking; she's still choking."

I gave her the phone numbers of three doctors to try until I got there. Putting down the phone, I saw before me the bewildered faces of the factory clerks. I scribbled down Clive's name and number and, thrusting it at them, blurted, "My little girl is choking. She's handicapped. Please keep trying this number and tell her father to go to the school right away."

As Mark and I raced to the car, I knew already that I was too late. I said, "Mark, Melanie is at school, and she's choking. Mummy's going to drive very, very fast, and you must stay in the back and hold on tight."

My beautiful 3-year-old boy got in the back and held on tight.

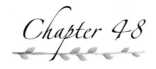

Chapter 48

THE WORST OF TIMES

How can I describe that drive? The Vita-Foam factory was in Mount Hope, at least 15 minutes drive from Woodbrook or 20 to 30 minutes away in traffic. It was 2 o'clock in the afternoon, and the Eastern Main Road was jammed.

I turned on the headlamps, pressed my hand on the horn, and drove past the double lanes of westbound traffic and through the red lights at Mount Hope, Mount Lambert, Petit Bourg. I reached the Croisee at San Juan, the most impossible of Trinidadian intersections, and sure enough, there was a huge tanker blocking the intersection.

I opened the door of the car, stood up, and screamed at the driver, "My child is dying; I have to get to her!"

Again a sea of shocked faces as the tanker moved aside, unquestioning.

The next task was to get over the Lady Young Road. I was out of the bumper-to-bumper traffic by then, but my old car was sluggish on this hill at the best of times. This was the worst of times, and as I pressed the accelerator to the floor, the engine struggling to respond, I knew once more that I was too late.

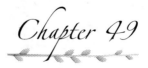

Chapter 49

THE END

Mercedes stood on the front step, her face the color of ash, with Melanie limp in her arms. "I got Dr. Roache; she said to meet her at Roxy roundabout."

As she leapt into the front seat and Sandra into the back, I could not look at Melanie. But as one limp arm brushed mine, I was overtaken by terror, and the voice that started screaming was mine, "She's cold, Mercedes. She's dead. It's over, it's over . . . ."

Dr. Roache was not at Roxy, and as the car reeled to a stop in front of her office some blocks away, Mercedes led the way into the building. Again, we saw the faces shaking their heads and saying, "She's gone to meet you at Roxy."

Back in the car, I could think only of the hospital and raced, horn once more blaring, past the St. James traffic to the Community Hospital at Cocorite.

Leaping out of the car, Mercedes rushed ahead, her arms filled with the beloved burden she would carry for the rest of her life.

I can only say that, throughout this terrible journey, I lost all the control that had kept me going through the wonderful years of knowing and loving Melanie. Mercedes ran ahead of me down the long polished corridor, but it was my screaming voice that led the way. Doors opened, and all at once, we were in a room with a doctor and some nurses.

I answered their questions about what had happened, and as they lay her on the bed, oxygen mask over her face, and started pumping her chest, I crouched in a corner some 6 feet away and waited, every ounce of belief and disbelief suspended for those few hopeful moments.

This was a doctor, he would save her.

Time was frozen for those moments. The doctor stopped, took off his stethoscope, and looked at me, shaking his head.

I screamed, "What, What is it? Is she dead? Tell me! Is she dead?"

As he nodded, I crouched on the floor, hearing that voice again, "No! It's not true! It can't be true! This is a dream, this is a dream, this is a dream...."

I went to the bed and took her into my arms. Time froze, the voice continuing. Then suddenly, the door opened and Dr. Camps walked in. I shouted at him, accusingly,

"Michael Camps! She's dead! She's dead!"

"What happened?"

"She choked," I said. "You remember how she nearly choked on the carrot? She choked on a piece of bread, and she's dead."

He said, "Give her to me," holding out his arms, and I said, "No!"

He said, "Just let me look at her," and took her out of my arms and laid her on the bed. As he examined her, the impossible hope flooded through me. But he said, "Yes, she's gone."

All at once my senses sharpened, and I saw several realities before me: the reality of my dead child on the bed, the reality of the resident doctor whose expression spoke his own uneasiness in the situation—a death on his hands of whose circumstances he knew nothing but for which he now had some responsibility. As I became aware of his dilemma, I was relieved to hear Dr. Camps explaining Melanie's problems to him, assuring him tacitly that there was nothing to be suspicious of in the circumstances of this death.

And then I looked, with new eyes, around the room. I saw before me the reality of Mercedes—the beautiful young woman who had become like my own daughter over the past year and who, with her playfulness and warmth, had brought such joy to Melanie. Mercedes stood silent and rigid against the far wall of the room, and I knew I had to share this experience with her. I had somehow to bring a measure of order and credulity to the unbelievable thing that had happened.

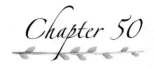

Chapter 50

SHE LOOKS ALL RIGHT

L
ooking back, I see that every moment of anxiety, of distress, of love and joy—every failure and every success with Melanie—had deepened my perception of the mystery that is life and prepared me for her death in such a way that I knew on the spot what my perspective must be.

As I called across the room to Mercedes, the words flowed easily as if they had been forever on the tip of my tongue. I reminded her how much she had loved Melanie and how much that love had been returned. Melanie died in the arms and in the care of someone she loved and trusted. She knew that she was not alone and that Mercedes was doing everything she could to help her. We had never deserted her. She had known that all her life. We had loved her unreservedly and had shown our love every day of her life.

Some weeks after her birth, my mother had asked a doctor in Jamaica to phone Dr. McDowall for his opinion on Melanie's condition. Dr. McDowall had said (I was not told this until years later) that he estimated that there was perhaps a 1% chance that she would survive infancy—1%!

"She could have died then, Mercedes, before we had a chance to know her, to love her. She could have come and gone like a ship in the night, and we would have lost her and never known what we had lost.

"But this way, we have gained. We have accomplished something. And she has gained. She gained a chance at life, and she gave it her very best. She had a life full of the kind of love some people never know in a long lifetime.

"We have nothing to regret, Mercedes, no fault to find, no guilt to bear, only the pain of losing her and we will have to live through that."

Mercedes could not cry, but I did; and as I looked at Melanie, as lovely in death as she had been in life, I knew that I was a totally different person than the one who had held her so shakily almost 6 years before.

Clive arrived and I had to repeat three times that she was dead before he heard what I had said.

He looked at her lying still in my arms and said, "But she looks like she's sleeping. She looks all right."

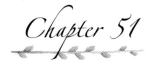

Chapter 51

GOODBYE

Philip's letter was read at the funeral and spoke for everyone who loved our beautiful Little Bird.

The news of your passing has brought many memories to mind, as well as much profound grief to me. When I remember the circumstances of your brief stay, I am amazed at the enormous impact you have made on our lives and the equally enormous legacy of lessons you have left with us. Although I am sad to think that I will never see you again, I am happy and proud to have been a part of your life, and find some consolation in the knowledge that you will continue to live in the lessons we have learned from you.

Your lessons are as extraordinary as the extraordinary love you received from your extraordinary parents. Your life is a tribute to their love and your lessons a blessing to the many who received them.

I am thankful for your life, and am with you today as much as your lessons are with me, forever.

In loving memory, Uncle Philip

EPILOGUE

I began writing this manuscript in Melanie's second year of life and completed it just before the first anniversary of her death. Twenty-seven years later, there is nothing in its telling that I would like to change. I see this account as simply a mother's story, whose appeal lies both in the uniqueness of its detail and the universality of its lessons.

On reading it, Clive said he remembered much of the story in a different way than I did. Undoubtedly, this is my story, perhaps even more than it is Melanie's. Mark, now 32, says he remembers the day I told him to hold on tight and stopped to scream at a truck that was blocking our way in the traffic. One day, in his teens, Mark brought me a picture of a beautiful teenaged girl modeling a summer dress in a magazine; he said, "Mum, doesn't this girl look just like how Melanie would've looked today?" She did, and I cried with joy that he had such a clear vision of his sister.

Melanie's memory lives on actively on both sides of our family. My brother, Philip, named his daughter Grace Melanie after her grandmother and her cousin. Robert, Melanie's brother from Clive's first marriage, named his daughter Abena, which was Melanie's second name.

Mercedes is a nurse in Trinidad and is married with two children. I believe that her experience with Melanie has enriched her life despite the terrible cloud it cast over her young adulthood.

I am a professor of special education at a university in the United States. My decision, 4 years after Melanie's death, to leave Trinidad, the Immortelle Center, and most important, my marriage, is probably related in part to the tremendous sense of emptiness that consumed me in the years after her death. I grieved intensely for about a year, and as I started to return to life, it was as if nothing I was doing engaged me sufficiently. The intensity Melanie had demanded left a vacuum that nothing I was then doing would satisfy. Since that time, the challenges of study, writing, work, and creating a new life have flowed into, if not filled, that vacuum. Both Clive and I remarried but retained a relationship marked by the bond of family. He and Mark continued to be, as it always seemed to me, like two peas in a pod.

Melanie's impact on my professional life has been immeasurable. My focus as a researcher and teacher of special education has been indelibly marked by my experience with her. In my teaching, I begin every course with a personal introduction that includes the lessons I learned from her, and I encourage undergraduate and graduate students alike to believe the messages of their hearts as they make professional decisions. In my research and writing, I try to represent the perspectives of parents—in particular, those whose voices have historically been underrepresented in the dialogue on disability. My commitment to this effort was deeply influenced by my growing perception of America's racial and socioeconomic divisions.

Consequently, my books have focused on these issues, as indicated by their titles:

- *Building Cultural Reciprocity with Families* (Harry, Kalyanpur, & Day, 1999)

- *Cultural Diversity, Families and the Special Education System* (Harry, 1992)

- *Culture in Special Education: Building Reciprocal Family–Professional Relationships* (Kalyanpur & Harry, 1999)

- *Why Are So Many Minority Students in Special Education? Understanding Race and Disability in Schools* (Harry & Klingner, 2005)

The Immortelle Center has been, for 2 decades, a nonprofit organization owned by the parents of students in the school and directed by Jackie Leotaud, whose daughter Raquel was the first pupil signed up for my little playgroup that became the Immortelle Center. In a society where limited public funding makes private and voluntary services essential, the Immortelle continues to offer shade to those who would wither in the unrelenting tropical sun. There are now two branches of the school—the second being a vocational training program and sheltered workshop for young adults with disabilities. Melanie's gift to her community lives on.

MELANIE

little girl
you blew my world apart
when you appeared
defying
with your intense fragility
my clean-cut classic image
of motherhood

but when you fixed those bright black
ackee-eyes on me
and clutched my heart with all your might
I knew
that it was sink or swim
for both of us

and so it was we swam against the tide
at one in strength and one inspiration

until you died
and blew my world apart
again

REFERENCES

Feurstein, R., Rand, Y., & Hoffman, M.B. (1979). *The dynamic assessment of retarded performers: The learning potential device.* Baltimore: University Park Press.

Finnie, N. (1975). *Handling the young cerebral palsied child at home.* London: Plume.

Harry, B. (1992). *Cultural diversity, families and the special education system. Communication and empowerment (Special Education Series).* New York: Teachers College Press.

Harry, B., Kalyanpur, M., & Day, M. (1999). *Building cultural reciprocity with families: Case studies in special education.* Baltimore: Paul H. Brookes Publishing Co.

Harry, B., & Klingner, J. (2006). *Why are so many minority students in special education? Understanding race & disability in schools.* New York: Teachers College Press.

Kalyanpur, M., & Harry, B. (1999). *Culture in special education: Building reciprocal family–professional relationships.* Baltimore: Paul H. Brookes Publishing Co.

Mahoney, G.J., & Seely, P. (1976). The role of the social agent in language acquisition. In N.R. Ellis (Ed.), *International review of research in mental retardation* (Vol. 8). New York: Academic Press.

READER'S GUIDE

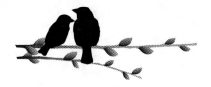

1. The book opens with Beth's frank admission of her fears following Melanie's birth as she looks at her new daughter and thinks about the challenges ahead: "You are beautiful, but if you're going to hang around and give me trouble, I'd rather you died." Are you shocked by this admission? Why do you think Beth chooses to be so brutally honest? How does this statement color your impressions as you read about Beth's intense commitment to her daughter's development?

2. In Chapter 16, *Initial Assessments,* Beth remarks that she remembers being surprised that the occupational and physiotherapist at the Ontario Crippled Children's Center were "On [Melanie's] side because they were positive and affectionate with Melanie, often saying, 'Good girl, Melanie.'" Beth's experience with medical personnel up to this point made her feel that they were not on Melanie's side. What are some things that professionals working with families of children with special needs can do to reassure parents that they are advocates for these children and their caregivers?

3. In Chapter 17, *Seeing,* Beth and Melanie first meet Dr. Karen Pape of the Sick Kids' Hospital Neonatology Department in Toronto. Beth remarks that it is "the spontaneity and freshness of [Dr. Pape's] approach that turned [her] mind around and taught [her] . . . how to look at a child as the child is without bias and preconceived notions." Without this "freshness of approach," Dr. Pape would have never made the remarkable observation of Melanie's attempt to compensate for lack of eye control by turning her head to view an object. Can you think of other situations in which a "freshness of approach" made (or can make) a difference in the family's understanding of their child's condition?

4. In Chapter 24, *The Turning Point,* Beth is told about some "extreme medical procedures . . . that could be used in an extreme case of failure to thrive." In a footnote, Beth describes how now (more than 25 years later) gastrostomies are common practice and her refusal to allow it "seems incomprehensible to special educators" today. Can you think of situations in which a family is left with only "extreme" choices? How can you better help them in their decision-making/coping process? How do you feel about Beth and the doctor's decision not to allow a gastrostomy?

5. How have the fields of early intervention and early childhood special education changed since Beth's search for services in the 1970s? How would you approach Melanie's case if you were the professional working with her today? What can still be improved upon when it comes to providing services for young children with severe disabilities and their families?

6. Nourishment is a major theme throughout the book, as Beth details Melanie's struggles to eat successfully and thrive across the different stages of her development. How does this elemental and basic skill affect the author's interactions with her daughter? In what ways does the author nourish Melanie beyond the physical act of feeding?

7. This book's roots took hold in the careful note-taking and observation the author undertook to chronicle Melanie's development. Beth worked diligently to record every detail to better inform Melanie's care and treatment, and this work evolved to become a powerful tribute to her experience and to her daughter. Was it Beth's experience as a loving mother or as an academic and professional that equipped her with such a careful eye for detail? Or was it both? What can professionals in early intervention and early childhood special education learn from Beth in terms of careful observation and record keeping?

8. How will reading about Melanie's story inform your interactions with children with special needs and their families?

9. In Chapter 30, *Seeking Another View,* Beth describes the "symbiotic" relationship that she had developed with Melanie.

She goes on to talk about how she would breathe with Melanie and could anticipate when Melanie was about to choke. How do you think this feeling of symbiosis between the mother and the child can aid in intervention? How can it hinder progress?

10. In Chapter 31, *The Forest or the Trees?*, Melanie is diagnosed with what turns out to be an inaccurate assessment of her condition. At the time, Beth questions her own role as a mother and what she sees in her child versus what she wants to see. How can professionals in early intervention reconcile the objective view of the outsider with the subjective view of the parent without being overly dismissive of either frame of reference?

11. When Beth first starts work at the Immortelle Center, one of her main hurdles is being able to adequately address the needs of all the children with varying disabilities. How do you approach intervention with each new child in terms of his or her unique physical, mental, and emotional needs, as well as those of the parents or caregivers? What are the pros and cons of grouping children with similar disabilities versus cross-grouping children of various ability levels?

12. At one point, Beth questions Melanie's progress, wondering if it is merely that she "learned it by heart" or if she truly understands the new words presented to her. She goes on to discuss how teachers of children with learning difficulties often "require many more demonstrations of their knowledge" than they would of typically developing children. She questions whether Melanie really did forget some things or, rather, whether she was simply fed up by the repetition! What are your thoughts on this idea?

13. Beth is very impressed with Sarah Blacha's handling of Melanie. It is in watching Sarah assume that Melanie understands a verbal direction that Beth realizes that her expectations and demands of Melanie were very low by comparison. What can professionals do to help parents not "aim too low" in an effort to avoid being disappointed by their child's progress? How can they ensure that parents do not expect too much?

14. Because of the time period in which Melanie was born, she did not receive a CT scan until she was 4 years old. Now, it's likely that Melanie would have had a CT scan much sooner. How would this have changed the course of her treatment? Do some research to think about the use of CT scans and other imaging technologies in developing treatment plans for children with disabilities.